D1388769

Comments on *Chronic Obstructive* *Primary Care* from readers

It provides a wealth of practical information for all health professionals who work in general practice.
Greta Barnes, Founder of the
National Respiratory Training Centre

This is an exceptional piece of work and one that I hope will be taken extremely seriously within Primary Health Care.
Lynn Young, Royal College of Nursing

I think that this is an extremely clearly written book, which is clearly going to be extremely important in highlighting the role of primary care in managing patients with COPD.
Michael Rudolf, Consultant Physician, Ealing Hospital

COPD in Primary Care really is excellent. I particularly like the logical layout of the text, making it easy to dip in and out and pick up the bits one is interested in.
E Neville, Consultant Physician St Mary's Hospital, Portsmouth

This is required reading for anyone involved in the multi-disciplinary approach to COPD Management. It is clear, concise and above all gives a common sense approach to this difficult but important problem.
Dr R N Harrison, Consultant Physician,
Respiratory Unit, North Tees and Hartlepool NHS Trust

It is without doubt the best book available for general practitioners who want a comprehensive account in chronic obstructive pulmonary disease.
Professor J J Reid, Head of the Department of General Practice,
University of Otago, New Zealand

Reviews of *Chronic Obstructive Pulmonary Disease in Primary Care*

Chronic Obstructive Pulmonary Disease in Primary Care

Fourth edition

All you need to know to manage COPD in your practice

Dr David Bellamy MBE, BSc, FRCP, MRCGP, DRCOG

GP with special respiratory interests in Bournemouth – recently retired. Trainer for Education for Health. Previous member of BTS and NICE COPD Guidelines groups

and

Rachel Booker RGN DN(Cert)HV

Respiratory Specialist Nurse and Freelance Medical Writer. Previously COPD Module Leader for Education for Health, Warwick. Previous member of BTS COPD Consortium

Class Publishing • London

The information presented in this book is accurate and current to the best of the authors' knowledge. The authors and publisher, however, make no guarantee as to, and assume no responsibility for, the correctness, sufficiency or completeness of such information or recommendation.

Printing history

First published 2000
Reprinted 2000
Second edition 2002
Reprinted 2003
Third edition 2004
Reprinted 2005; with amendments 2006
Fourth edition 2011

The authors and publisher welcome feedback from the users of this book. Please contact the publisher:

Class Publishing Ltd,
The Exchange, Express Park, Bristol Road, Bridgwater TA6 4RR
Telephone: 020 7371 2119
Fax 020 7371 2878 [International +4420]
Email: post@class.co.uk
Website: www.class.co.uk

A CIP catalogue record for this book is available from the British Library

ISBN 978 185959 225 0

Designed by Martin Bristow

Typeset by Mach 3 Solutions Ltd

Indexed by Valerie Elliston

Line illustrations by David Woodroffe

Printed and bound in Great Britain by Good News Digital Books, Stevenage, Herts

Contents

Foreword to the fourth edition

by Dr Michael Rudolf FRCP
Consultant Physician Ealing Hospital
Chair, NICE COPD Guideline Development Group

In the seven years that have passed since publication of the third edition of this book, enormous advances have been made in our understanding of what constitutes good management of COPD. These include not only improvements in our knowledge of basic mechanisms (encompassing the concept of COPD as a systemic disease with important co-morbidities) and how to use effective therapies, but also other crucially important areas such as earlier diagnosis, multidimensional assessment, and key features of new guidelines and strategies.

It is a pleasure to acknowledge that David Bellamy and Rachel Booker have been meticulous in incorporating all these, and many other, important topics into this new edition, which appears at a time when both the organisation of the British National Health Service and the commissioning of services are undergoing enormous changes. Never has there been a greater need for a comprehensive account of how best to look after people with COPD in primary care, and this book admirably fulfils that role.

The information and advice given by the authors on virtually every aspect of COPD management should be required reading for anyone involved in the care of people with COPD, and not necessarily confined to those working in primary care. The fourth edition of this important book provides a sound basis for ensuring continuous improvements in the standards of care that our patients with COPD deserve.

Foreword to the first edition

by Greta Barnes MBE

Founder of the National Respiratory Training Centre

In recent years alterations in health care and health policy have accelerated change in the management of chronic diseases such as diabetes, asthma and hypertension. There has been an increasing shift of emphasis from secondary to primary care, and a collaborative approach has been encouraged not only between hospital and general practice but also between GP and practice nurse.

By 2020 chronic obstructive pulmonary disease (COPD), the 'smokers' disease', is likely to become the UK's fifth most common cause of death. It will also be managed chiefly in the community. At present it has been acknowledged that COPD is not widely understood by the vast majority of doctors and nurses, particularly in primary care. Many patients may have been misdiagnosed and therefore inappropriately treated.

The publication of Chronic Obstructive Pulmonary Disease in Primary Care has proved very timely. It gives a wealth of practical information for all health professionals who work in general practice. The authors highlight the importance of correct diagnosis and the value of spirometry as well as how to treat and manage the patient with COPD. The chapter on smoking cessation, which is the single most important intervention, provides invaluable advice to the reader, as does the section on ways to improve the quality of life for patients with this debilitating condition.

David Bellamy and Rachel Booker have a wealth of experience looking after COPD patients in general practice. In this book they have demonstrated the value of combining medical and nursing experience so that they can help others strive for excellence.

Undoubtedly this book will attract a wide range of health professionals who work in the community. It will also serve admirably to complement Education for Health's Chronic Obstructive Pulmonary Disease Training Programme.

The authors are to be congratulated on producing a much-needed book – the first of its kind for primary care.

Foreword to the first edition

by Professor Peter Calverley MB, FRCP, FRCPE
Professor of Medicine (Pulmonary and Rehabilitation),
The University of Liverpool

Chronic obstructive pulmonary disease is a common, often unrecognised, source of morbidity and mortality in the UK and throughout the world. Traditionally, it has been seen as a 'dull' condition devoid of exciting symptoms or physical signs that help enliven the teaching of medical students and largely unresponsive to treatment. This therapeutic failure on the doctor's part is often excused by the recognition that the condition itself is usually brought on by cigarette smoking and therefore is 'the patient's own fault'. This has led to a type of therapeutic nihilism, which can no longer be justified given the changes in our understanding of the causes and consequences of COPD as well as the availability of more effective

treatments. Despite encouraging reductions in the use of cigarettes, especially by middle-aged men, the problems of the COPD patient persist and are likely to do so even in the developed economies of the world. Patients who might have succumbed from their illness had they continued smoking in the past now develop symptoms related to their previous lung damage as they age, and this respiratory disability is an increasing burden to all those involved in the care of older patients. We now have the techniques relatively readily available to help make a firm diagnosis of COPD and to distinguish these patients from the many others with a bewildering array of similar symptoms produced by different pathologies, where the therapeutic approach and the likely prognosis will vary. The management of the COPD patient is increasingly multidisciplinary and the patients themselves are entitled to explanations not only of how their disease arises but also what the different treatments recommended do and what kind of improvement they are likely to achieve. The dilemma for health professionals is that this type of information has often not been available to them during their training, nor is it sufficiently up to date to help them form a useful management plan. This book has set out to remedy these problems.

This short book provides a wealth of information and practical advice, based on clinical experience and evidence-based recommendations. It is written by a general practitioner and a nurse educator, both with wide experience of respiratory disease and who are familiar with the kinds of questions that someone new to this field is bound to ask. They stress the importance of a positive diagnosis and of a positive therapeutic approach. When the correct patients are identified, useful things can be done for them even if this is unlikely to completely abolish all their symptoms once the disease itself is advanced.

The authors have been keen to demystify the role of pulmonary function testing while indicating how it fits into everyday clinical management. Their recommendations are up to date, and include some of the very latest clinical trial data as well as practical comments about the management of complications and acute exacerbations of disease. The result is a handbook of practical information that will be helpful to everyone concerned with this common clinical problem.

Hopefully, those who read and use this book will feel more confident about managing COPD in their daily practice, which in turn will begin to reverse the expectations of patients and doctors that, in the past, have been so low but no longer need to be quite so pessimistic.

Acknowledgements

We thank Greta Barnes, Founder of the National Respiratory Training Centre, and Richard Harrison, consultant respiratory physician at Stockton on Tees. Without their encouragement, this book would never have been started.

We also thank both our families for their support and tolerance.

Abbreviations

AHR airway hyper-responsiveness

AMP adenosine monophosphate

BMI body mass index

BTS British Thoracic Society

CT computed tomography

FEV$_1$ forced expired volume produced in the first second

FEV$_1$/FVC% the ratio of FEV1 to FVC, expressed as a percentage

FVC forced vital capacity – the total volume of air that can be exhaled from maximal inhalation to maximal exhalation

IL interleukin

JVP jugular venous pressure

LRTI lower respiratory tract infection

LTOT long-term oxygen treatment

MDI metered dose inhaler

NE neutrophil elastase

NOTT Nocturnal Oxygen Therapy Trial

NRT nicotine replacement therapy

NSAID non-steroidal anti-inflammatory drug

OSA obstructive sleep apnoea

PaCO$_2$ arterial carbon dioxide tension

PaO$_2$ arterial oxygen tension

PDE phosphodiesterase

PEF peak expiratory flow – the maximal flow rate that can be maintained over the first 10 milliseconds of a forced blow

RV residual (lung) volume

TLC total lung capacity

TLCO diffusing capacity for carbon monoxide, or diffusing capacity

TNF tumour necrosis factor

VC (relaxed or slow) vital capacity

Introduction

Main points

1 Chronic obstructive pulmonary disease (COPD) is a common and important respiratory disorder that causes considerable morbidity and patient suffering.

2 It comprises a spectrum of diseases, including chronic bronchitis, emphysema, long-standing asthma that has become less responsive to treatment and small airways disease.

3 COPD is a chronic, slowly progressive disorder characterised by airflow obstruction that varies very little from month to month.

4 The main cause of COPD is cigarette smoking.

5 COPD is more common in men and with increasing age: 2% of men aged 45–65 and 7% of men over 75 years. Some 28,000 people die from COPD each year in the UK.

6 It results in a large economic burden to the nation, in excess of £1 billion per year for health care.

7 The symptoms of breathlessness and coughing increasingly affect levels of activity, work, lifestyle and social interaction.

8 The current British Guidelines on COPD come from the National Institute for Health and Clinical Excellence (NICE). They were first published in 2004 and were updated in 2010.

9 Other guidelines around the world have also been updated, including a new version of the global guidelines, GOLD, produced jointly by the National Heart, Lung and Blood Institute (NHLBI) and the World Health Organization (WHO), and combined American Thoracic Society and European Respiratory Society Guidelines.

10 The Department of Health has produced a National Clinical Strategy on COPD, setting out policies for best clinical practice. This was, published as a consultation document in 2010.

What is new in this fourth edition

Since the first edition of this book was published in 2000, Chronic Obstructive Pulmonary Disease (COPD) has gained a much greater prominence in both primary and secondary care, resulting in improved standards of diagnosis and patient management. COPD was considered a disease for which little could be done other than to stop patients smoking. New developments, a National Strategy, updated NICE Guidelines and greater awareness and interest have contributed to a very much more positive attitude and a holistic approach to care, from early diagnosis to end of life. Patients are correctly placed at the centre of decisions on disease education, treatment and self-management.

The volume of research relating to COPD has increased hugely and pharmaceutical companies are searching for better and new forms of treatment. This increased enthusiasm is very appropriate as COPD is undoubtedly one of the most common and important chronic diseases, causing a large burden of symptoms to patients and a major workload and economic burden to health services around the globe. Unlike many other chronic diseases such as coronary artery disease, the number of sufferers with COPD worldwide is increasing.

One of the new innovations in Primary Care in the UK has been the introduction of the Quality and Outcomes Framework (QOF) for a range of chronic diseases, including COPD and asthma. This has greatly encouraged practices to correctly identify and diagnose patients with COPD and to try to differentiate it from chronic asthma. Importantly, it has firmly placed spirometry as the gold standard for diagnosis. The current QOF criteria follow the NICE COPD and Scottish Intercollegiate Guideline Network/British Thoracic Society (SIGN/BTS) Asthma Guideline advice for diagnosing airflow obstruction, and use the criteria of an increase in FEV_1 (forced expired volume in the first second) of more than 400ml to strongly suggest asthma. The recommended use of post-bronchodilator measurements will help to exclude COPD in some borderline patients and alert practitioners to the possibility of asthma.

From 2009 the QOF criteria include measuring the MRC dyspnoea index, which is important in assessing patient disability. QOF is an excellent start, but in future this needs to become much more patient care orientated, looking more at clinical outcomes, with inclusion of important clinical markers such as the number of exacerbations per year.

In 2010 the Department of Health published a consultation on a National Clinical Strategy (formerly called a National Service Framework – NSF) for COPD. This evidence-based document complements clinical guidelines and sets out quality requirements and strategies for best clinical practice. More attention is paid to early disease detection, improving access to care and providing uniform quality of care throughout the country. It should raise the profile of COPD to a much wider lay and professional audience and improve overall standards of patient care. The Clinical Strategy is fully discussed in Chapter 12.

Since the last edition the international GOLD Guidelines have been updated several times and NICE also updated their Guideline in 2010. One current area of hot discussion is which spirometric criteria to adopt to define most accurately airflow obstruction. To provide international uniformity and continuity with the National Strategy, NICE has adopted the GOLD classification of COPD severity based on FEV_1 % predicted levels and the FEV_1/FVC ratio. GOLD uses primarily the FEV_1/FVC ratio that, if below 0.7, suggests airflow obstruction. However, the normal range of the ratio decreases with age and, in older patients the lower limit is more in the range of 0.65. Hence, using the ratio alone over-estimates COPD in the elderly.

There is also some doubt as to the extent that patients found to be at GOLD stage 1 (an abnormal ratio plus a FEV_1% above 80% predicted), unless symptoms are present, represent any real form of lung disease. NICE has made this point in their guideline revision. Assessing prevalence using GOLD stage 1 doubles the numbers of patients diagnosed with COPD compared with the old NICE criteria for mild disease (FEV_1/FVC below 0.7 and FEV_1 predicted less than 80%). A more accurate alternative option, which is gaining popularity, is to adopt normal predicted levels based on the lower limit of the normal range (LLN) – those spirometric values for FEV_1, FVC and FEV_1/FVC ratio which fall outside the 5th percentile for a normal population. It is likely that new Guidelines will adopt this measure in the future and spirometer manufacturers incorporate the calculations in new machines.

In the past few years it has become increasingly apparent that COPD is a multi-system disease that affects not only the lungs but also many other parts of the body, from skeletal muscles and bones, to the heart and blood. It also causes significant anxiety and depression in a high proportion of patients. COPD is linked with other important chronic diseases such as coronary heart disease, heart failure, diabetes and lung cancer. Inflammatory mechanisms may be linked in some of these disorders and there is also a common trigger factor in cigarette smoking.

Awareness and knowledge of COPD both in the general public and the healthcare sector are still inadequate. Major improvements have occurred but there is still much to do.

Why COPD is important

Chronic obstructive pulmonary disease (COPD) is one of the most common and important respiratory disorders in primary care. About 28,000 people die from COPD each year in the UK, and the disease results in considerable morbidity, impaired quality of life, time off work, and more hospital admissions and GP consultations than asthma. In the past, COPD management was seriously neglected and the only treatment offered was to stop smoking. Since the end of the 1990s we have seen considerable improvements, with a much better understanding of diagnosis and the range of treatments available. Continuing better education of the public and healthcare professionals is the key to further raising standards of care.

COPD is a spectrum of diseases that includes:

- chronic bronchitis,

- emphysema,

- long-standing asthma that has become less responsive, with limited reversibility to treatment,

- small airways disease.

The unifying feature of COPD is that it is a chronic, slowly progressive disorder characterised by airflow obstruction that is not fully reversible and varies very little from day to day and month to month.

COPD is caused mainly by cigarette smoking. The risk of COPD is increased by a factor of 10–14 in active smokers compared to non-smokers. In the UK smoking is attributed as the main cause of COPD in 87% of males and 84% of females. A recent Danish study has shown that over 25% of people who smoke over a 20-year period will develop COPD. There are still no clear pointers as to what makes this 25% susceptible to tobacco smoke. It is probable that there are genetic factors that increase susceptibility to smoking but as yet no definite chromosomal abnormalities have been identified, other than the fairly rare alpha-1 antitrypsin deficiency. Family studies have found that siblings of people with emphysema are three to four times more likely than controls to develop COPD if they smoke.

Once COPD has been diagnosed stopping smoking is the only effective way of slowing disease progression. Recent clinical trials such as TORCH and UPLIFT are providing some evidence that drug therapy may have some beneficial effects on mortality, although the data did not quite reach statistical significance. The earlier in the disease progression this occurs the better the result. COPD cannot be cured but much can be done to improve symptoms and quality of life.

Acute exacerbations are now seen to have a very adverse affect on patient symptoms and, if frequent, can accelerate overall decline. Many therapies have been shown to reduce exacerbation frequency as well as improving symptoms.

Pulmonary rehabilitation can result in major benefits in mobility and well-being but is still not widely available. Long-term oxygen therapy and some forms of surgery can prolong life.

The 1990s saw great improvements in the management and organisation of asthma treatment in primary care. COPD, by contrast, was largely ignored and rightly dubbed the 'Cinderella respiratory disorder'. This situation began to change with the publication and widespread dissemination to GPs and practice nurses of the British Thoracic Society (BTS) *COPD Guidelines* in December 1997. Since then, interest and research have steadily increased worldwide. Many other Guidelines have been published and updated. The international GOLD Guidelines in their 2006 update list the following goals of management:

- relieve symptoms

- prevent disease progression

- improve exercise tolerance

- improve health status

- prevent and treat complications

- prevent and treat exacerbations

- reduce mortality.

Guidelines are important in providing an evidence-based rationale for accurate and appropriate clinical decision making. However, their information is not useful unless successfully disseminated to all primary care doctors and nurses in a simple, readily digestible format. Respiratory champions for each PCT need to set up educational networks to disseminate the content of Guidelines and the new Clinical Strategy.

How important is COPD?

The current prevalence of COPD in the UK, based on QOF figures, is between 1.5% and 2% with considerable regional variations. It is estimated that there are 3 million people suffering from COPD but only 900,000 people have been currently diagnosed and are receiving treatment. These 'missing millions' need to be found and given smoking advice and symptomatic treatment before their disease becomes too severe.

Men are more likely to be affected than women, but in some European countries there are no gender differences in prevalence rates. The frequency of COPD increases with age with prevalence rates of 2% in men aged 45–65 years and 7% in men over 75. The prevalence rates for women are rising more rapidly than men. This is in part related to the change in their smoking habits since the 1970s and it also appears that women are more susceptible to tobacco smoke. Women who smoke are estimated to be 13 times more likely to develop COPD than a non-smoker.

In 2004 COPD accounted for 5% of deaths in men and 4% in women in the UK. Mortality tends to be greater in urban areas, particularly in South Wales, the north-west of England and Scotland. There is a strong association with lower social class and poverty that can be explained only partly by the higher smoking rates of this group.

The milder stages of COPD are often relatively symptom free and patients have little need to consult a GP. There is also a known reluctance for patients with mild symptoms of breathlessness and smoker's cough to seek help as they are relatively unconcerned about mild symptoms of gradual onset. They may acknowledge that smoking is the likely cause of their symptoms, but do not wish to be told that they need to stop smoking. Thus many patients first present with moderate stage disease. The high proportion of undiagnosed patients is a major hurdle to detecting and treating early disease, where it has the greatest benefit to prevent disease progression. A recent UK study found that over 80% of patients found to have airflow obstruction reported no respiratory diagnosis. Even in those found to have severe COPD only 47% reported any diagnosed respiratory disease.

The whole issue of screening for early detection of COPD remains controversial, with argument surrounding studies that have found little or only modest increases in smoking cessation when at risk, asymptomatic smokers are found to have airflow obstruction. The case finding method used in the van Schayck study looked at smokers or ex-smokers over 35 years with one or more respiratory symptoms. In those with a cough, 28% were found to have airflow obstruction – a high yield. The new Clinical Strategy sets out an extensive programme for screening and performing spirometry in at-risk children and young adults, as well as a case finding programme for smokers over 40 years. This will involve a symptom-based questionnaire to provide an initial screen to identify those on whom to perform spirometry. Results of pilot studies are awaited, but funding for such major projects is, at present, likely to be limited.

It is never easy to persuade smokers to quit but if successful at an early stage of the disease, most will not develop symptomatic COPD. This will produce major personal benefits for them as well as significant cost saving to the NHS.

The global situation

The WHO estimates that 600 million people have COPD worldwide. More than 2.5 million die of the disease each year, which is about the same as HIV/AIDS. In 2001, COPD was the fifth greatest cause of death in developed counties and sixth in under developed countries; by 2020 WHO estimate it will have moved up to third place. COPD is the tenth leading cause of disease related disability.

Over the past few years there have been some major, high-quality surveys performed in various countries around the world as part of the Burden of Lung Disease (BOLD) initiative. The reported prevalence of COPD is much greater than previously reported, but there is considerable variation between countries. The prevalence of stage 2 GOLD COPD severity or higher (equivalent to the NICE mild COPD category) was 10.1% overall, 11.8% for men and 8.5% for women. Age was not, surprisingly, an important contributory factor with an odds ratio (OR) of 1.94 increase prevalence for every 10 years of age. The risk with increasing tobacco consumption was OR 1.28 in women and 1.16 for men for every extra 10 pack years smoked.

Looking at causes of COPD worldwide can paint a different picture to the high percentage linked to smoking in the UK. WHO estimates that in high-income countries, 73% of COPD mortality is related to smoking, with 40% related to smoking in nations of low and middle income. Exposure to dusts, vapours or fumes in the workplace was estimated in a USA study to account for COPD in 19.2% of cases, with the figure being even higher in never smokers at 31.1%. This finding is likely to be even more important in under developed nations.

Globally, one of the most important risk factors might be exposure to biomass fuels, such as wood, straw, animal dung and crop residues, used to heat and cook in poorly ventilated homes. Biomass fuels are used in approximately 50% of homes worldwide. This equates to 3 billion people exposed to indoor smoke from biomass fuels. WHO estimates that, for lower income countries, 35% of people with COPD develop the disease from this cause. This is particularly so in women in rural areas. Much needs to be done to educate, improve ventilation and convert to safer fuels.

The increasing number of co-morbid chronic diseases associated with COPD contribute to disability and early mortality. Deaths in COPD are often attributed to other causes such as cardiovascular disease, lung cancer and other causes.

What is the economic burden of COPD?

The current total cost of COPD to the NHS is likely to be in excess of £1 billion, the most recent data being in 2003 when the estimate was £980 million. Secondary care management accounts for over half the total, with the figure for hospital admissions in 2003 being £530 million for the UK. Since 2000, admissions to hospital have increased by 50%.

In an average health district serving 250,000 people there will be 14,500 GP consultations every year. The average cost per patient per annum is £810.42, at least three times the cost of a patient with asthma. Of this figure, 54.3% is due to in-patient care, 18.6% for treatment, 16.4% for GP contact, 5.7% for A&E visits and 5% for tests. Not surprisingly, the cost per patient dramatically increases with disease severity from £150 per year with mild disease, to £308 with moderate disease and £1,307 with severe disease.

A typical COPD patient consults 2.4 times per year, and has an estimated mean annual drug bill of £124. Oxygen therapy is an expensive part of therapy. There have been many changes in prescribing criteria and suppliers in the past few years with more rational use of oxygen concentrators. However, oxygen cylinders are still too widely prescribed, particularly for short burst use, which research tells us is of no benefit.

Patients with severe COPD have frequent exacerbations – 2–3 per year. These are a common reason for hospital admission. A survey in Merseyside calculated that 12.5% of all medical acute admissions were for exacerbations of COPD. In an average health district the annual inpatient bed days amount to 9,600, compared with 1,800 for asthma. The length of stay is notably longer than for asthma: 10 days for COPD compared with 3.6 days for asthma. Hospital admission for COPD has a sinister effect on prognosis, with 15% mortality within 3 months and 25% within a year.

COPD also causes considerable loss of time from work – 24 million days in 1994/5. The economic cost for that period amounted to £600 million in state benefits. Adding the value of lost work to employers brings the total economic cost to the nation to a staggering £2.7 billion in 2004!

Doctors' and patients' attitudes to COPD

Historically, the medical profession had a negative attitude to COPD, but this has changed significantly. Many practice nurses have had specific training in COPD care and performing spirometry, and effectively conduct annual or more frequent reviews on patients. Patients are being more fully educated and encouraged to self manage. In hospitals there are more focused units for COPD admissions and greater use of Hospital at Home schemes. Despite these advances there are still problems that need resolving.

- There are still many GP practices where interest levels in COPD are low.

- Although much more spirometry is being performed in primary care there are concerns about the technical quality of these recordings and the fact that some staff have little accredited training.

- There is need for greater knowledge on spirometry interpretation.

- There are missed opportunities for identifying new patients.

The public are generally poorly informed about COPD and even when symptoms are present, people seem reluctant to see their GP about the condition. A survey conducted on behalf of the British Thoracic Society's COPD Consortium in 2001 interviewed 866 adults about their knowledge of COPD and its symptoms. Only 35% had heard of the term 'COPD', although 92% had heard of chronic bronchitis and 79% had heard of emphysema. Just under 30% of the sample had experienced breathlessness on mild exertion and 22% frequent winter coughs and colds. When symptomatic people were asked if they had visited a GP with these symptoms only 54% said yes. The reasons given by 65% of them were that they were either not bothered by the symptoms or were unaware they needed to be checked by a doctor. Another 23% said they would not go to the surgery, as the GP would just tell them to stop smoking. A further 21% were too busy.

The data from this survey highlight the considerable obstacles there are to finding and diagnosing the early stages of the disease.

Identifying patients

People with or at risk of COPD can be identified by the following measures.

- Performing spirometry on smokers or ex smokers over 35 years, who have any of the symptoms of exertional breathlessness, chronic cough, regular sputum production, frequent winter bronchitis, or wheeze.

- Reviewing patients over 35 labelled as having asthma or those taking bronchodilators who also smoke.

- Evaluating patients with an existing diagnosis of chronic bronchitis, emphysema or COAD

- The Department of Health needs to do more to educate the general public and encourage them to report to primary care earlier when symptoms appear.

What can be done?

GPs and practice nurses can considerably improve the symptoms and lifestyle of patients with this very common disease. By making a correct diagnosis as early in the disease process as possible, maximum influence can be brought to bear on the patient to stop smoking and thus prevent the development of severe and disabling symptoms.

Once the disease is manifest, patients should be given the opportunity to have optimal bronchodilator therapy – the most important treatment to improve breathlessness and exercise tolerance. Patients with significant disability (MRC dyspnoea grade 3 or higher) should be considered for pulmonary rehabilitation as it can result in major benefits. As COPD progresses and exacerbations occur inhaled steroids need to be added and other medication proven to reduce exacerbation frequency considered. Patients should be provided with a self-management action plan to treat exacerbations as early as possible. The adverse social and psychological effects of the disease need to be recognised, carefully assessed and, where possible, alleviated. Patients with more severe disease may need to be referred to hospital for assessment for long-term oxygen, bronchodilators via nebuliser or possible surgery.

In the past the approach to managing COPD has been too negative. Much can be done for these patients, and primary care is the main site for their diagnosis and treatment. This book aims to equip you, as a primary care professional, to achieve this. NICE has put the COPD patient at the centre of management and decision-making.

In 2003 the Respiratory Alliance, a group representing primary and secondary care, nurses and patient groups, produced a report on improving high-quality integrated respiratory care called *Bridging the Gap*. In it they set out the following 'reasonable expectations' for patients with COPD.

- All smokers have the right to co-ordinated smoking cessation services.

- They have the right to timely and accurate diagnosis.

- They have the right to management in line with approved guidelines.

- They have the right to access pulmonary rehabilitation services from an early stage in their disease.

- They have the right to access appropriate secondary care services.

- They have a right to appropriate assessment and practical support for the use of supplementary oxygen.

- They have a right to integrated health, social and palliative care services.

Further reading

Respiratory Alliance (2003) *Bridging the Gap – commissioning and delivering high quality integrated respiratory healthcare.* Respiratory Alliance, Direct Publishing Solutions, Cookham, Berks

Buist AS, McBurnie MA, Vollmer WM, et al. (2007) International variation in the prevalence of COPD (The BOLD study): a population-based prevalence study. *Lancet* **370**: 741–50

British Thoracic Society (2006) *Burden of Lung Disease.* 2nd edn. Available at http://www.brit-thoracic.org.uk/library-guidelines/bts-publications/burden-of-lung-disease-reports.aspx

British Lung Foundation (2003) *Casting a shadow over the nation's health.* Lung Report III. Available at http://www.lunguk.org/OneStopCMS/Core/CrawlerResourceServer.aspx?resource=8F2B9E63-09F9-49F6-BD8B-FB788E62627B&mode=link

Healthcare Commission (2006) *Clearing the Air. A national study of Chronic Obstructive Pulmonary Disease.* Available at www.healthcarecommission.org.uk

British Lung Foundation (2005) *COPD Resource Pack for Primary Care Organisations.* Available at http://www.lunguk.org

Department of Health (2010) *Consultation on a strategy for services for Chronic Obstructive Pulmonary Disease (COPD) in England.* Available at www.orderline.dh.gov.uk

Enright P (2008) The use and abuse of office spirometry. *Primary Care Respiratory Journal* **17**: 238–42

British Lung Foundation (2005) *Femme Fatality The rise and rise of COPD in women*. British Lung Foundation, London

Mannino DM, Buist AS (2007) Global burden of COPD: risk factors, prevalence, and future trends. *Lancet* **370**: 765–73

Global Initiative for Chronic Obstructive Pulmonary Disease (2009) *Global Strategy for the Diagnosis, Management and Prevention of Chronic Obstructive Pulmonary Disease*. Available at www.gold-copd.com

National Clinical Guideline Centre (2010) Chronic Obstructive Pulmonary Disease: the management of chronic obstructive pulmonary disease in adults in primary and secondary care. London. CG101. Available at http://guidance.nice.org.uk/CG101/Guidance/pdf/English

Salvi S, Barnes P (2010) Is exposure to biomass smoke the biggest risk factor for COPD globally. *Chest* **138**: 3–5

van Schayck CP, Loozen JM, Wagena E, et al. (2002) Detecting patients at high risk of developing chronic obstructive pulmonary disease in general practice; cross-sectional case-finding study. *British Medical Journal* **324**: 1370–4

Main points

1 COPD is an umbrella term that includes the pathological processes of emphysema, chronic bronchitis, small airways disease and chronic asthma.

2 The most important risk factor is cigarette smoking.

3 Treating persistent asthma early and aggressively with inhaled steroids may reduce the development of chronic airflow limitation.

4 Chronic mucus production alone is not always associated with the development of progressive airflow limitation; however, when there is progressive airflow limitation, chronic mucus production may accelerate the decline in lung function.

5 Emphysema is thought to develop as a result of an imbalance between elastase and anti-elastase activity in the lung.

6 Loss of lung elastin, such as occurs in emphysema, contributes to airway collapse, particularly during exercise.

7 Hyperinflation of the lungs leads to increased breathlessness on exertion.

8 Disruption of gas exchange leads to polycythaemia, cor pulmonale and respiratory failure.

9 COPD is associated with systemic inflammation and effects in parts of the body outside the lungs; skeletal muscle, bones, heart and blood.

COPD is not a single pathological entity, but an overlapping syndrome of the four main conditions:

1 emphysema
2 chronic bronchitis
3 small airways disease
4 chronic asthma.

It has thus defied definition in terms of pathology. NICE defines COPD as:

> 'characterised by airflow obstruction and the condition is predominantly caused by smoking. The airflow obstruction is usually progressive, not fully reversible and does not change markedly over several months.'

GOLD guidelines similarly define COPD in functional terms but both GOLD and NICE also allude to the underlying pathological process and its cause. GOLD defines COPD as:

> 'a disease state characterised by airflow limitation that is not fully reversible. The airflow limitation is both progressive and associated with an abnormal inflammatory response of the lungs to noxious particles or gases.'

Some patients have an asthmatic element to their COPD and it will be possible to reverse their airflow obstruction to some degree. However, even when this is the case, the lung function *cannot be returned to normal*, no matter how intensive the treatment.

Risk factors

Cigarette smoking

Cigarette smoking is overwhelmingly the most important risk factor for the development of COPD. Indeed, this is reflected in the GOLD and NICE guidelines' definition of the disease. Although COPD can occur in non-smokers, about 87% of cases in the UK are thought to be a direct result of cigarette smoking.

Lung function declines after the age of 30–35 years as part of the ageing process (Figure 2.1).

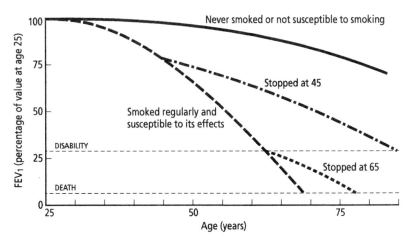

Figure 2.1 The decline in lung function as part of the normal ageing process
and as accelerated by cigarette smoking.
(Reproduced, with permission, from Fletcher and Peto, 1977)

- In normal, healthy non-smokers the rate of decline of FEV_1 is about 25–30ml a year.

- In 'at-risk' smokers the rate of decline may be double that, at about 50–60ml a year – and some smokers decline even faster than this.

Why some smokers are at risk of this accelerated decline and others are not has been the subject of considerable research. Involvement of genetic factors is suggested by the 'clustering' of COPD cases in some families. Although some of this increased risk may be due to shared environmental factors, studies of diverse populations suggest that shared environment does not provide a full explanation. The search for a 'COPD gene' has revealed a number of possible candidates, but has so far been inconclusive.

What is known is that lung function declines steadily over the years of smoking but the FEV_1 often drops below 50% of predicted before symptoms appear. Patients usually present with symptoms of COPD between the ages of 50 and 70 years.

Although lost lung function is not regained when smoking is stopped, the rate of decline returns to that of a non-smoker or non-susceptible smoker (see Figure 2.1). This study by Fletcher and Peto (1977) highlights the importance of detecting such high-risk smokers early, and persuading them to stop smoking. If they can be persuaded to stop, they may never suffer from severe, disabling and symptomatic COPD.

The large US Lung Health study shows similar positive results for stopping smoking. The main findings were:

- The rate of decline of FEV_1 over 5 years was 31ml/year in quitters versus 62ml/year in continued smokers

- Younger quitters benefitted a little more than older quitters

- Women improved more than men but female smokers deteriorated more rapidly

- Heavy smokers benefitted more than lighter smokers.

However, whatever the baseline lung function there was still an improvement.

A further major study published in 2009 (Kohansal et al.), based on the Framingham population database, followed a much more diverse population than Fletcher and Peto. Baseline age ranged from 13 to 71 years and average follow-up time was 23 years. The main findings were that healthy, never-smoker females achieve full lung growth earlier than males and their rate of decline with age was slightly lower (but not significantly) – 17.6ml/year versus 19.6ml/ year. Smoking increased the rate of decline in both sexes – 38.2ml/ year in males and 23.9ml/year in females. Previous respiratory symptoms at baseline enhanced decline. Quitting smoking reduced the rate of decline at all age groups and if quitting occurred before the age of 30, the rate of decline assumed that of never smokers.

Thus, even when a smoker has developed symptomatic disease, stopping smoking will still result in worthwhile salvage of lung function and improved life expectancy. The main message for patients is:

It is never too late to stop!

Passive smoking

Most non-smokers are exposed to environmental tobacco smoke (ETS). Exposure can be high in children and in the socially disadvantaged. For adults the main risk of exposure is living with a smoker. ETS was estimated to have caused 12,200 deaths in the UK in 2003, most of which were related to exposure in the home.

There have been a number of large epidemiological studies looking at the effect of ETS on the risk of COPD in non-smokers. A meta-analysis of eight studies, largely involving exposure from a spouse, showed an excess risk of 25%. Other studies have shown a small but significant decrease in lung function in passively exposed non-smokers. It is estimated that for those living with a smoker 2,700 die of disorders due to passive smoking in the age group 20–64 per year, and 8,000 per year in the over 65 age group.

In China, where smoking has become an epidemic, a study on ETS exposure, both at home and in the workplace, showed an increased risk of COPD with an OR of 1.48.

In the hospitality industry the risk of COPD is greatly increased. A recent study estimates that 617 people in the industry die as a result of exposure to smoke (all causes) each year. The ban on smoking in the workplace and public places will hopefully do much to reduce exposure to ETS in these locations. A Childrens' Charter has just been launched to try to protect children from tobacco smoke exposure in the home and also in cars.

Increasing age

COPD is a slowly progressive disorder and becomes considerably more common in older age. There are at least three times as many patients with COPD over 65 years as there are below 65, with prevalence rates of 2% in men aged 45–65 years and 7% in men over 75. Symptoms appearing in someone under the age of 40 years should be regarded with suspicion and investigated fully because COPD is unlikely to be the cause, unless the sufferer is deficient in alpha-1 antitrypsin (α_1-AT). This is discussed in more detail later.

Gender

COPD is currently more common in men than women in the UK. A 1997 study of physician-diagnosed COPD showed a prevalence rate of:

- 1.7% of men
- 1.4% of women.

This is widely acknowledged to under-estimate the true prevalence of the disease. A modelling exercise, based on the Health Survey for

England (2001) estimates the overall prevalence of COPD to be 3.1% of the English population (3.9% of men and 2.4% of women). It should be remembered that this model does not include the COPD 'hot spots' in South Wales and Scotland. The other bad news is that, although the prevalence increased in men by 25% between 1990 and 1997, the increase in women during the same period was 69%. In men the prevalence of COPD levelled out in the mid-1990s but is continuing to rise in women.

The differences between male and female smokers might be related to the fact that, in this age cohort, smoking was more common in men than in women. With the increase in the number of women smokers, the preponderance of males is changing. Some recent work has suggested that female smokers are at even greater risk of developing COPD than their male counterparts.

The large, Copenhagen City study followed over 8,000 men and women with initial normal lung function for 25 years. At the end of the study the percentage of men with normal lung function ranged from 96% of never smokers to 59% of continuous smokers. For women the proportions were 91% and 69% respectively. The 25 year incidence of moderate and severe COPD was 20.7% and 3.6% respectively, with no apparent differences between men and women. The absolute risk of developing COPD among continuous smokers is at least 25%. This is a much higher figure than the 15% quoted in Fletcher and Peto's study from the 1970s. The Copenhagen patients were older and it is suggested that perhaps smokers become progressively more susceptible to smoke as they grow older.

Airway hyper-responsiveness

Airway hyper-responsiveness (AHR) has been proposed as a risk factor for the development of COPD. Certainly AHR is not the sole preserve of the person with asthma. It has been demonstrated extensively in smokers. Smokers also have raised levels of IgE, the antibody associated with atopy and asthma.

This observation forms the basis of the so-called Dutch hypothesis. Some doctors in the Netherlands have long regarded COPD and asthma as two aspects of the same process, and believe that at-risk smokers share an 'allergic' constitution that, when combined with smoking, is expressed as COPD. However, this hypothesis is controversial and it has been argued that raised levels of IgE and increased AHR in COPD patients could be the *result* of smoking rather than a pre-existing factor.

Lower socio-economic status

The prevalence of COPD is highest among people in lower socio-economic groups. Smoking rates are higher in these groups, but this may not be the sole causative factor.

Low birth weight is associated with a reduced FEV_1 in adult life. Airways develop in the first 16 weeks of gestation, and alveoli mature and increase in number in the last six weeks of gestation and first three years of life. The number of alveoli reaches adult levels of about 300 million by the age of 8 years. Thus, malnutrition of the fetus and serious lower respiratory tract infection (LRTI) in infancy during these periods of lung development may result in lung function failing to reach full potential. This may be an independent risk factor for reduced lung function in adult life and increased risk of COPD.

Maternal smoking has been extensively linked with low birth weight and recurrent LRTI in infancy, as have poor housing and social deprivation.

Poor diet

It has been suggested that antioxidants in the diet protect against the harmful effects of smoking and that a low dietary intake of antioxidant vitamins, such as vitamin C, is associated with decreased lung function and increased risk of COPD. A recent large US study has shown that in men, a diet rich in fruit, vegetable and fish has about half the risk of developing COPD compared with a diet of refined grains, red meat, desserts and chips.

Poor diet is also associated with socio-economic deprivation.

Occupation

Certain jobs have been linked with COPD. Coal mining is probably the most well-recognised occupational risk factor, but cotton processing, farming and other dusty occupations may also be relevant, particularly when added to the effects of smoking. Welding fumes are highly toxic, and welding, particularly in confined spaces, is suspected of being a risk factor. However, in the UK at present the only occupational cause of COPD for which compensation may be paid is coal mining.

Air pollution

Air pollution is often blamed by COPD sufferers for their disease. Before the Clean Air Acts of the 1950s, urban dwelling was associated with an increased risk: the air was polluted with heavy particles, soot and sulphur oxides. The pollution now experienced is mainly from vehicle exhaust emissions and photochemical pollutants such as ozone, produced by the action of sunlight on exhaust fumes. It is seldom disputed that these are respiratory irritants and that episodes of high pollution are associated with increased hospital admissions for respiratory problems. The role of these irritants *as a cause* of COPD, however, is more controversial. Nowadays, urban dwelling in the UK does not seem to pose a greater risk of COPD than rural dwelling.

Biomass fuels

Globally about 50% of households and 90% of rural households use solid fuels – coal and biomass – as the main domestic source of heating and cooking. The combination of harmful effects from these combustion products and poor home ventilation cause prolonged adverse exposure, particularly for women and children. The WHO estimates that globally 1.6 million deaths per year can be attributed to indoor smoke from solid fuels. It ranks indoor air pollution as the 10th most preventable risk factor causing burden of disease, and in developing countries it is the fourth most important.

Wood smoke is a particular problem, either unprocessed or as charcoal, with animal dung and crop residues also posing a risk. In developing countries, particularly India, SE Asia, China, Latin America and Africa, almost 50% of deaths from COPD could be attributed to biomass fuels and about 75% of these occur in women. Many of these women are never smokers. Biomass fuel smoke increases the risk of COPD 2.3 times, which is similar to the risk from smoking and alpha-1 antitrypsin deficiency. There is an additive effect in those who also smoke, with the risk rising to 4.4 times.

Interventions include encouraging cooking outdoors, improvements in household ventilation and stoves and better, cleaner fuels.

Deficiency of alpha-1 antitrypsin

A rare, but well-recognised, risk factor for COPD is the inherited deficiency of alpha-1 antitrypsin. This is a protective enzyme that counteracts the destructive action of proteolytic enzymes in the lung. Deficiency of it is associated with the early development – between the ages of 20 and 40 years – of severe emphysema (see also the section 'Emphysema', below). The deficiency is inherited in a homozygous fashion with a frequency of 1:4000 of the population. The possession of a single abnormal chromosome does not seem to cause severe disease, but may still increase susceptibility to COPD and may also be associated with liver disease. There is usually a strong family history of COPD. Family members should be tested for alpha-1 antitrypsin deficiency and, if affected, must be very strongly advised never to smoke.

Genetics

Alpha-1 antitrypsin deficiency is an extensively studied genetic risk factor for COPD. It is now believed that many other genetic factors increase (and decrease) an individual's risk of developing COPD. Why there seem to be familial clusters of COPD cases, and why some smokers develop COPD and others do not, has intrigued many researchers. The genetics of COPD is being investigated intensively.

Chronic asthma

The diagnosis of asthma is based on the recognition of a characteristic pattern of symptoms and signs and the absence of an alternative explanation for them. The key is a careful history.

- More than one of the following symptoms: wheeze, breathlessness, chest tightness and cough, particularly if:
  - Symptoms worse at night and early morning
  - Symptoms in response to exercise, allergen exposure and cold air
  - Symptoms after taking beta-blockers or aspirin
- History of atopic disease

- Family history of asthma and/or atopic disease

- Widespread wheeze heard all over the chest

- Otherwise unexplained low FEV_1 or PEF

- Otherwise unexplained blood eosinophilia.

Long-standing asthma may result in permanent damage to the airways and subsequent loss of reversibility of airflow obstruction – the key feature of asthma. Long-standing bronchial hyper-reactivity can cause hypertrophy of the bronchial smooth muscle, just as skeletal muscles will hypertrophy if exercised regularly. Chronic epithelial disruption may result in the deposition of collagen in the basement membrane and fibrosis of the sub-mucosal layer. The end result is a narrowed and distorted airway that can no longer bronchodilate fully.

The duration and severity of the asthma are risk factors for the development of fixed airflow obstruction. Approximately 1 in 10 people with early-onset asthma will develop a degree of fixed airflow obstruction; for those with late-onset asthma the proportion is higher – around 1 in 4. Smoking considerably increases this risk.

Recent studies have suggested that early intervention with inhaled steroids reduces the risk. Work in children with persistent asthma has shown that a two-year delay in introducing inhaled steroids results in a reduced potential for the lung function to improve, compared with the improvement found in children who commenced inhaled steroids immediately. Further work with adults has shown similar results, suggesting that early diagnosis and early, aggressive treatment with inhaled steroids may reduce the risk of long-term chronic airflow obstruction. There are also implications for ensuring that patients adhere to the therapy they are prescribed and don't smoke.

Occupational asthma – particularly if the diagnosis is delayed and exposure prolonged – can lead to chronic persistent symptoms and fixed airflow obstruction, even after the patient is removed from the offending occupational sensitiser.

Chronic bronchitis

Chronic bronchitis is defined by the Medical Research Council as:

'The production of sputum on most days for at least three months in at least two consecutive years.'

This definition describes a set of symptoms that are extremely common, if not universal, among long-term smokers and widely recognised as the 'smoker's cough'. Not all smokers whose illness fits the definition of chronic bronchitis will have an accelerated decline in lung function; between 75% and 85% of smokers do not, after all, develop COPD. However, the GOLD guidelines and the National Clinical Strategy suggest that those with a persistent cough and sputum production and a history of exposure to risk factors should be considered 'at risk' and should be tested for airflow obstruction even if they do not complain of breathlessness. Research from the Netherlands has supported this suggestion. Random testing of smokers aged between 35 and 70 years revealed a reduced FEV_1 in 18% of all smokers. The percentage with a reduced FEV_1 rose to 27% in smokers with cough and to 48% of smokers over 60 years who also had a cough.

Mucus in the airways is produced by mucus glands, situated mainly in the larger airways, and by goblet cells, found mainly in the lining of the smaller airways. Mucus glands produce about 40 times more mucus than the goblet cells. Goblet cells are normally absent from small airways and their presence there defines a condition associated with smoking; mucus metaplasia. Excess mucus in large airways can be cleared by coughing but mucus in the small airways can not. It may be that the excess mucus production in smokers not affected by progressive airflow obstruction reflects changes in the large airways. This chronic hypersecretion of mucus with little airflow obstruction, in the absence of other reasons for chronic mucus production such as bronchiectasis, is known as 'simple bronchitis'. However, in at-risk smokers who are developing chronic airflow obstruction, excess mucus production seems to accelerate the rate of decline of their lung function.

Chronic production of mucus is unpleasant and may predispose the sufferer to lower respiratory tract infection, but on its own is not thought to be universally associated with the development of airflow obstruction. Excess production of mucus ceases in the majority of smokers when they stop smoking, although an initial short-term increase is a common experience in smokers when they quit.

Emphysema

Emphysema is defined in structural and pathological terms as:

> *'A condition of the lung characterised by abnormal, permanent enlargement of the air spaces distal to the terminal bronchiole, accompanied by destruction of their walls.'*

This definition describes a destructive process that is largely associated with cigarette smoking. Cigarette smoke is an irritant and results in low-grade inflammation of the airways and alveoli. Bronchoalveolar lavage of smokers' lungs reveals increased numbers of inflammatory cells, notably macrophages and neutrophils. These inflammatory cells produce elastases – proteolytic enzymes that destroy elastin, the protein that makes up lung tissue. In health, these enzymes are neutralised by anti-elastases, anti-proteolytic enzymes, the most widely studied of which is alpha-1 antitrypsin. Figures 2.2 and 2.3 show the histology of normal lung tissue and of emphysema.

Alpha-1 antitrypsin deficiency accounts for 1–2% of all cases of diagnosed COPD. It provides a good model for our current understanding of the role of elastases and anti-elastases in the development of emphysema.

In early experiments, elastases introduced into lung tissue deficient in alpha-1 antitrypsin digested that lung tissue, thus producing emphysema. When alpha-1 antitrypsin was introduced into the deficient lung tissue – thereby effectively making it 'normal' – it protected the lung against the action of the elastases and thus prevented emphysema.

That elastases are responsible for the destruction of lung tissue was confirmed by further experiments. A purified elastase was derived from neutrophils, a white blood cell attracted into the lungs of smokers. This neutrophil elastase (NE) was instilled into the lungs of experimental animals, causing a transient decrease in lung elastin, which then gradually returned to normal. However, although the loss of elastin was temporary, the structure of the animals' lungs was permanently damaged.

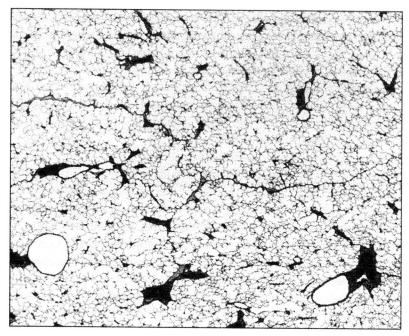

Figure 2.2 The histology of normal lung tissue

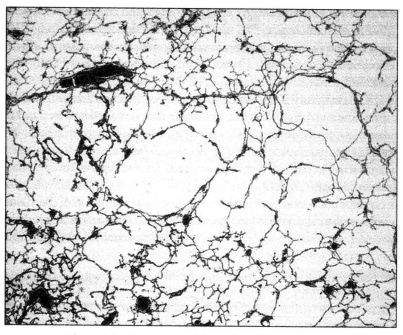

Figure 2.3 The histology of lung affected by emphysema

Although these and other experiments helped to explain the mechanisms behind the development of emphysema in people who are deficient in alpha-1 antitrypsin, it remains less clear what happens in people who are not deficient in this anti-proteolytic enzyme. There are several theories but further investigation is needed.

One theory is that, in some smokers, excessive numbers of inflammatory cells are attracted into the lungs in response to the irritant effects of cigarette smoke. These inflammatory cells, particularly neutrophils, are responsible for the release of elastases into the lung tissue; if too many are attracted into the lung, the amount of elastase they produce may outstrip the protective capacity of the anti-elastases. It is thought that in some individuals the inflammatory cells themselves produce excessive amounts of elastases.

The elastase/anti-elastase hypothesis for the development of emphysema in humans is that the irritant effect of cigarette smoke increases the level of elastases in the lungs beyond the body's ability to neutralise them. Over many years lung elastin is lost, lung tissue is destroyed and emphysema results.

Yet another hypothesis is that there is excessive inactivation of the protective anti-elastases such that the individual is somewhat deficient in these protective enzymes. It is thought that this inactivation may be caused by oxidants that are both present in cigarette smoke and released from the activated inflammatory cells present in the airways of smokers.

In practice, all these mechanisms may be interacting in a single individual.

Elastases, NE in particular, have been implicated in the development of chronic bronchitis as well as emphysema. They have been found to produce an increase in the number of goblet cells, a feature of chronic bronchitis. NE is also a potent inducer of mucus secretion, and causes a reduction of ciliary beat frequency.

Thus elastase/anti-elastase imbalance may be implicated not only in the development of emphysema but also in the pathogenesis of chronic bronchitis.

These hypotheses can be summarised as:

- Abnormally high numbers of inflammatory cells are attracted into the airways, resulting in excessive production of elastases.

- The inflammatory cells in the airways produce abnormally large amounts of elastases.

- Oxidants found in cigarette smoke and released from inflammatory cells inactivate the protective anti-elastases in the lung.

Small airways disease

Cigarette smoking may result in pathological changes in the small airways as well as the alveoli. Structural changes in the small airways 2–5mm in diameter have been found in young smokers who have died suddenly from causes other than respiratory disease. Cigarette smoke causes chronic inflammation in the airways and repeated cycles of inflammation and repair. This leads to remodelling of the tissues of the airways. The changes include:

- inflammation and oedema

- fibrosis

- collagen deposition

- smooth muscle hypertrophy

- occlusion of airway with mucus.

As a result, the airway becomes narrowed and distorted, causing resistance to airflow. Unfortunately, there can be considerable change in these airways without giving rise to symptoms. Indeed, this level of the bronchial tree is often referred to as the 'silent area' of the lungs.

COPD – a mixed spectrum of diseases

Although we can recognise the pathological entities of chronic bronchitis, small airways disease and emphysema, it is usual, clinically, for COPD patients to have features of more than one. It is also important to remember that COPD is not simply a disease of the lungs. It is increasingly recognised that COPD produces systemic inflammation and effects throughout the body – on muscle, bones, the heart and blood. These effects are covered in detail in the next chapter.

Consequences

Narrowing of the bronchioles results in increased resistance to airflow. Loss of elastin in the alveolar walls in emphysema contributes to the collapse of the small airways. The lung parenchyma is made up of the walls of alveoli, which support the small airways in the same way that taut guy ropes hold open the walls of a tent. Destruction of the alveolar walls in emphysema means that this support is lost and the airways will tend to collapse (Figure 2.4). Airway collapse is exacerbated by forced exhalation, such as occurs on exercise, and air is trapped in the lungs. Patients with emphysema may naturally adopt a strategy that helps to 'splint' the airways open. 'Pursed-lip' breathing helps maintain air pressure in the small airways, preventing them from collapsing. Patients seem to be 'grabbing' air and 'paying it out' gently. It is a useful, though not universal, clinical sign.

The elastic walls of the alveoli provide some of the driving force behind exhalation. Loss of this elasticity causes the lungs to become 'floppy' and hyperinflated. Emphysematous lungs may be 2–3 litres bigger than normal, but most of this extra capacity is inaccessible. Hyperinflation causes the diaphragms to flatten and the accessory muscles of respiration are then used to aid respiration. The inefficient respiratory movements caused by hyperinflation lead to

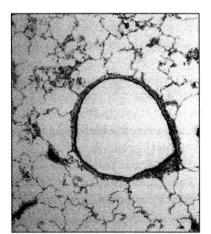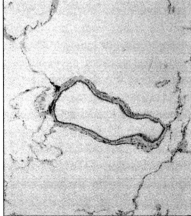

Figure 2.4 Histology showing the loss of the 'guy ropes', resulting in airway collapse

increased breathlessness on exertion, when the work of breathing is heightened and the respiratory rate is raised.

Loss of the alveolar/capillary interface causes disruption of gas exchange. The surface area for gas exchange in normal lungs is about the size of a tennis court. Emphysema reduces this area and thus reduces the capacity to exchange oxygen and carbon dioxide in the lungs. In the early stages of the disease the body is able to compensate for this loss by increasing the respiratory drive. As the disease progresses, however, the ability to compensate successfully diminishes and the blood gases become persistently abnormal, with serious consequences.

When the respiratory drive is responsive, abnormalities of blood gases will result in an increase in both respiratory drive and respiratory rate. The blood gases will be normalised but the patient will be breathless. Eventually the progression of the disease overcomes the ability of even the most responsive respiratory drive to compensate, and respiratory failure ensues.

Breathlessness makes everyday activities such as shopping, cooking and eating difficult. Weight loss is common and is associated with a poor prognosis. It was originally thought that weight loss in COPD was due to a combination of increased expenditure of energy at rest, because of the increased effort of breathing, and difficulty in maintaining an adequate energy intake. It is now recognised that weight loss in COPD is more complex and that systemic inflammatory processes are a major component.

Loss of lean body mass affects the ability to fight infection. Infective exacerbations may become more common and recovery will be slower. (Weight loss and nutrition are discussed in more detail in Chapters 3 and 10.)

Some patients seem to have a less responsive respiratory drive and, as the disease progresses, they will become unable to normalise their blood gases. They will be less breathless but will suffer from the long-term consequences of low levels of oxygen in the blood (hypoxia), cor pulmonale, pulmonary hypertension and polycythaemia.

Polycythaemia A way for the body to adapt to chronic hypoxia is to produce more haemoglobin to carry what little oxygen is available, increasing the number of erythrocytes and raising the packed cell volume (haematocrit). However, this predisposes an already less mobile patient to deep vein thrombosis and pulmonary embolism.

Pulmonary hypertension and cor pulmonale As the severity of COPD increases and blood oxygen levels drop, a series of complex changes may occur in the pulmonary arterial vessels. Hypoxia is a potent pulmonary vasoconstrictor causing rises in pulmonary artery pressure. Once established this is infrequently fully corrected by oxygen therapy. A persistently raised carbon dioxide level also acts as a vasoconstrictor.

In patients with COPD and hypoxia changes occur in the peripheral pulmonary arteries, with thickening of the intima layer with new muscle cells. This results in blood vessel narrowing and increased pressure. Destruction of lung tissue, which occurs in emphysema, can result in hypoxia for various reasons. It may cause a mismatch of ventilation and blood perfusion to areas of lung, thus reducing the potential for gas exchange in those lung areas. It may also reduce the blood flow to some alveoli from gas trapping and thus increase the pressure within the alveoli. Patients with secondary polycythaemia have increased blood viscosity and this may also contribute to pulmonary hypertension. Pulmonary hypertension often acutely worsens with exercise.

For a simplistic but helpful analogy for hypoxic pulmonary capillary constriction, imagine the lungs as a railway station. To work efficiently, passengers (*oxygen*) must reach the platforms (*alveoli*) where the trains (*blood supply*) can pick them up. If the passengers cannot reach the platforms (*poor ventilation*), the trains will go away empty and the railway system will be inefficient (*ventilation/perfusion mismatch*). If this situation persists, the railway line will be shut down (*pulmonary capillary constriction*). Eventually the track will be lifted so that, even if the passengers do reach the platform, the trains will no longer be there to pick them up. (*Structural changes in the blood vessel walls eventually result in irreversible capillary constriction.*)

Pulmonary hypertension is common in severe COPD and may be found in up to 40% of patients. It is not easy to recognise clinically and progresses slowly but, once established, it carries a poor prognosis. The right ventricle has to work harder to pump blood through a network of narrowed, constricted and disrupted pulmonary arterial vessels. This initially may cause hypertrophy of the ventricle, leading to muscle dysfunction. Eventually the ventricle fails, with the development of peripheral oedema. This syndrome is termed cor pulmonale. It is akin to right heart failure, but the latter can result from a range of causes, including problems with the left ventricle. Cor pulmonale increases in prevalence with the severity of COPD and occurs in 40% of patients with a FEV_1 below 1L and 70% of those with an FEV_1 below 0.6L. The development of oedema is usually a late feature and may first appear acutely during an exacerbation. The clinical pictures described above are recognisable as the 'pink puffer' and the 'blue bloater', but such terminology is out of favour and not particularly helpful. In practice the picture is less clear and patients often cannot be placed neatly into one or other category. Suffice it to say that some patients with appalling lung function and intolerable breathlessness will struggle on with reasonable blood gases whilst others, with less severely impaired lung function, will develop oedema and cor pulmonale relatively early. Intermittent ankle oedema and central cyanosis are a poor prognostic sign. Untreated, the three-year survival of such patients is only 30%. Long-term oxygen therapy (LTOT) can increase survival considerably. Cyanosis can be difficult to detect clinically and monitoring of oxygen saturation with a pulse oximeter in primary care will help early identification of patients who may benefit from LTOT. A saturation of less than 92% when the patient is well should prompt referral for oxygen assessment. The use of oxygen in COPD is covered in detail in Chapter 10.

Further reading

Risk factors

Agertoft L, Pedersen S (1994) Effects of long-term treatment with an inhaled corticosteroid on growth and pulmonary function in asthmatic children. *Respiratory Medicine* **88**: 373–81

Barker DJP, Godfrey KM, Fall C et al. (1991) Relation of birth weight and childhood respiratory infection to adult lung function and death from chronic obstructive lung disease. *British Medical Journal* **303**: 671–5

Buist AS, Vollmer WM (1994) Smoking and other risk factors. In: Murray JF, Nadel JA (eds) *Textbook of Respiratory Medicine.* WB Saunders, Philadelphia PA; 1259–87

Fletcher C, Peto R (1977) The natural history of chronic airflow obstruction. *British Medical Journal* **1**: 1645–8

Haahtela T, Jarvinen M, Kava T et al. (1994) Effects of reducing or discontinuing inhaled budesonide in patients with mild asthma. *New England Journal of Medicine* **331**: 700–5

Hu G, Zhou Y, Tian J, et al. (2010) Risk of COPD from exposure to biomass smoke. A meta analysis. *Chest* **138**: 20–30

Kohansal R, Martinez-Camblor P, Agusti A et al. (2009) The natural history of chronic airflow obstruction revisited. *American Journal of Respiratory and Critical Care Medicine* **180**: 3–10

Lebowitz M (1977) Occupational exposures in relation to symptomatology and lung function in a community population. *Environmental Research* **44**: 59–67

Lebowitz MD (1996) Epidemiological studies of the respiratory effects of air pollution. *American Journal of Respiratory and Critical Care Medicine* **9**: 1029–54

Lokke A, Lange P, Scharling H et al (2006) Developing COPD: a 25 year follow up study of the general population. *Thorax* **61**: 935–9

Mann SL, Wadsworth MEJ, Colley JRT (1992) Accumulation of factors influencing respiratory illness in members of a national birth cohort and their offspring. *Journal of Epidemiology and Community Health* **46**: 286–92

O'Connor GT, Sparrow D, Weiss ST (1989) The role of allergy and non-specific airway hyperresponsiveness in the pathogenesis of chronic obstructive pulmonary disease. *American Review of Respiratory Disease* **140**: 225–52

Royal College of Physicians (2005) *The medical case for clean air in the home, at work and in public places. A report on passive smoking by the Tobacco Advisory Group of the Royal College of Physicians.* Royal College of Physicans, London

Schwartz J, Weiss ST (1990) Dietary factors and their relation to respiratory symptoms. *American Journal of Epidemiology* **132**: 67–76

Silverman EK, Speizer FE (1996) Risk factors for the development of chronic obstructive pulmonary disease. *Medical Clinics of North America* **80**: 501–22

Soriano JR, Maier WC, Egger P et al. (2000) Recent trends in physician diagnosed COPD in men and women in the UK. *Thorax* **55**: 789–94

Torres Duque C, Maldonado D, Perex-Padilla R, et al. (2008) Biomass fuels and respiratory diseases. A review of the evidence. *Proceedings of the American Thoracic Society* **5**: 577–90 van Schayck CP, Loozen JMC, Wagena E (2002) Detecting patients at high risk of developing chronic obstructive pulmonary disease in general practice: a cross-sectional case-finding study. *British Medical Journal* **324**: 1370–4

Varraso R, Fung TT, Hu FB, et al. (2007) Prospective study of dietary patterns and chronic obstructive pulmonary disease among US men. *Thorax* **62**: 786–91

Pathology

MacNee W (1995) Pulmonary circulation, cardiac function and fluid balance. In: Calverley P, Pride N (eds) *Chronic Obstructive Pulmonary Disease*. Chapman and Hall Medical, London; 243–91

Peto R, Speizer FE, Moore CF et al. (1983) The relevance in adults of airflow obstruction, but not of mucous hypersecretion in mortality from chronic lung disease. *American Review of Respiratory Disease* **128**: 491–500

Stockley RA (1995) Biochemical and cellular mechanisms. In: Calverley P, Pride N (eds) *Chronic Obstructive Pulmonary Disease*. Chapman and Hall Medical, London; 93–133

COPD as a systemic disease, co-morbidity and cause of death

Main points

1 COPD should be considered as a systemic disease and not one purely affecting the lungs.

2 Raised levels of inflammatory markers such as CRP, TNF-α, and Interlukins IL-6 and IL-8 have been found in the blood of COPD patients, levels increasing with COPD severity.

3 COPD increases the risk of developing other diseases such as cardiovascular disease and lung cancer, and metabolic disorders such as diabetes.

4 The chronic inflammation associated with COPD may help to explain associated systemic problems such as muscle wasting, osteoporosis and anaemia.

5 Reduced lung function (FEV_1) is an independent risk factor for mortality, on a parity with the risk of raised cholesterol.

It has been known for some time that COPD is associated with chronic inflammatory changes in the lung and this is believed to play a central role in the pathogenesis of the disease. There is now an increasing body of evidence to suggest that COPD is also linked with systemic inflammation.

Smoking alone is also associated with inflammation in the lower airways and with systemic inflammation. The earliest changes in smokers are increased numbers of alveolar macrophages – cells that ingest smoke particles. Such change may reverse with quitting smoking and could be a body defensive mechanism.

As COPD develops there are increases in the number of neutrophils, CD8 T-lymphocytes and macrophages in the lung. During exacerbations the number of these cells greatly increases and they may be joined by eosinophils. This pattern of inflammation is different to that seen in asthma.

35

Systemic clinical manifestations, such as muscle wasting and weight loss are often seen in patients with COPD. The mechanisms for such changes are not clear but may be linked to increased numbers of neutrophils and levels of inflammatory markers found in the blood, including C-reactive protein (CRP), fibrinogen, tumour necrosis factor (TNF)-alpha, and interleukins IL-6 and IL-8. Such inflammatory markers are also found in conditions such as rheumatoid arthritis, where muscle wasting can also be a feature. Increasingly impaired lung function is significantly correlated with elevated levels of inflammatory markers. Patients with severe COPD have higher levels of CRP and TNF-alpha, which in turn is related to lower Body Mass Index (BMI) and decreased muscle mass. Systemic inflammation also appears to be related to an accelerated decline in lung function and is increased during exacerbations.

Reduced FEV$_1$ and increased mortality

A study in Renfrew and Paisley in Scotland in the mid-1990s (Hole et al. 1996) found that people with a FEV$_1$ below 73% of the predicted value had almost twice the level of all cause mortality compared with those who had normal lung function. The study made adjustments for smoking, blood pressure, BMI and cholesterol. The risk for ischaemic heart disease was 1.56 times greater for men and 1.88 for women; 2.53 and 4.37 respectively for death from lung cancer and 1.66 for both sexes for stroke. This and subsequent studies have calculated that having reduced lung function is a greater predictor of all cause and cardiac mortality than a raised cholesterol. Sin et al. (2005), using a lower FEV$_1$ predicted value of 63%, found a five fold greater risk of death from ischaemic heart disease compared to those with normal lung function.

The same research group (Gan et al. 2004) have correlated levels of the same systemic inflammatory markers as above with reduction in FEV$_1$. They found that a low FEV$_1$ more than doubled the chance of an elevated CRP. Smoking on its own also increased these markers and, with both a reduced FEV$_1$ and smoking, the effect was additive, increasing the risk three fold. The combination of COPD and a raised CRP increases the risk of myocardial infarction.

The effects of systemic inflammation on arteries are still not clear, but in studies of the cause of death in COPD patients, up to a half die of cardiovascular disease.

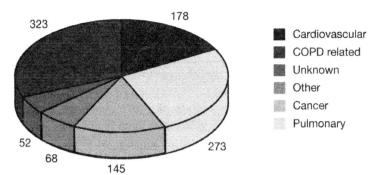

Figure 3.1 Causes of death in COPD patients – FEV 1 <50% predicted. Reproduced from the TORCH study with permission from GSK.

COPD mortality – what is the cause of death?

It would be logical to anticipate that most patients with COPD would be likely to die from a respiratory cause. However, a review of the literature by Sin et al. (2006) shows that other causes play a major role. In many studies cardiovascular causes contribute up to 40% and cancer, particularly lung cancer, may lead to almost a third of deaths. When patients have severe COPD many more die of respiratory failure. Figure 3.1 shows the distribution of causes of death from the recent large TORCH study. These patients had more severe COPD at the start of the study and consequently there is a higher proportion of pulmonary related deaths.

The nature of the causal pathways between these conditions is poorly understood, but there is good evidence that COPD is a risk factor for lung cancer and that COPD may precede cardiovascular mortality.

Co-morbid conditions associated with COPD

The following diverse conditions are associated with COPD.

- Cardiovascular disease
- Lung cancer
- Skeletal muscle wasting

- Osteoporosis

- Metabolic syndrome, diabetes

- Hormonal disturbances

- Anaemia

- Anxiety and depression.

As patients age they often develop more than one chronic disease and, indeed, it is estimated that at least 50% of people over 65 years have three or more chronic diseases. Smoking is a common risk factor to many of the above but there is evidence to suggest a link with COPD as a separate causative trigger. The pathological mechanisms suggested have been many, particularly systemic inflammation, hypoxia, increased oxidative stress and genetic predisposition, but there are no very clear proven links. Probably the important message is to no longer consider COPD as a disease solely of the lungs.

Cardiovascular

A range of cardiovascular conditions are more common in COPD patients. As we have already discussed, reduced FEV_1 is an independent predictor of dying from a myocardial infarction. The increased risk of cardiovascular disease includes myocardial infarct (1.89), hypertension (1.6), chronic heart failure (3.75), atrial fibrillation (1.98), pulmonary embolism (2.72) and stroke (1.33). The most likely link is the presence of low grade systemic inflammation in COPD and atherosclerosis, which could drive both pathologies.

Arterial stiffness – a good predictor of cardiovascular events – is found more often in patients with COPD and is perhaps linked to the level of low grade inflammation. Treatment with statins in patients with COPD exacerbations significantly improved survival. More formal studies are needed to evaluate fully the potential benefits of statins in this situation.

Lung cancer

Moderate and severe COPD increase the risk for lung cancer 2–5 fold compared with incidence rates in smokers without COPD. Lung cancer is also more common in people with COPD who have never smoked. Decrease in lung function is a strong predictor of lung cancer mortality and women seem to be more susceptible to developing cancer where reduced lung function is present.

There may be some genetic links to susceptibility for developing COPD and lung cancer. Treatment of COPD with inhaled steroids does not reduce lung cancer mortality.

Skeletal muscle wasting

Muscle wasting is commonly present in COPD and results in muscle weakness, exercise intolerance and impaired quality of life. The muscle changes in COPD are a form of myopathy that involves a spectrum of metabolic changes. Muscle wasting is increased with accelerated protein breakdown. This is thought to be linked to inflammatory cytokines such as TNF-α and interleukin 6. Other factors such as inactivity and hypoxia are contributory to muscle wasting. Exacerbations of COPD will also have an adverse effect on muscle function.

Osteoporosis

Osteoporosis is more common in COPD. In one study of untreated COPD patients osteoporosis was found in 28% of patients compared with 0% in age matched controls. Over half the patients recruited for the TORCH study (moderate and severe COPD) had osteoporosis or osteopenia. A survey of 465 COPD patients and a control group assessed the prevalence of vertebral deformities – unreported clinical fractures – and found deformities in 31% of COPD patients and 18% of controls.

The risk of osteoporosis increases with greater severity of COPD. Women seem more affected than men. When treatment with high dose inhaled and oral steroids is commenced there may be additional risk. It would seem prudent therefore to assess bone mineral density in all severe COPD patients and treat with bisphosphonates according to treatment guidelines.

Metabolic conditions

Obesity appears more common in COPD and with it the risk of metabolic syndrome and diabetes (relative risk 1.5–1.8). Many of the patients have a shift from fat free tissue to fat mass, although this is also a trend of ageing.

Hormonal changes

Male patients have been found to have lower testosterone levels and there is a greater risk of hypogonadism. This is relevant as, if present, it may contribute to muscle wasting. There is also impairment of growth hormone function, which may also have an adverse effect on muscles.

Anaemia

Many chronic disorders result in a normochromic anaemia. This is often termed 'anaemia of chronic disease'. COPD can now be added to the list.

Anaemia is present in a surprising 13–17% of COPD patients, presumably linked to chronic inflammation. Anaemia is independently associated with increased breathlessness and reduced exercise capability. Treatment of anaemia with blood transfusion under clinical trial conditions improved breathing but is not a clinical treatment option. Erythropoetin is unlikely to be a treatment as there is end organ resistance to it and iron supplements may be detrimental.

Of interest, polycythaemia, a more well-known secondary effect of COPD, was found in only 6% of patients and was not related to any functional symptoms.

Anxiety and depression

These are common in COPD and often are not diagnosed and treated. The prevalence varies between 10% and 42% for depression and 10–19% for anxiety. Risk is higher with increasing COPD severity, being greatest at 62% in patients on long-term oxygen therapy, and also after exacerbations. Depression significantly impairs quality of life, reduces physical activity and affects family life. There are also adverse effects on treatment adherence, increased frequency of hospital admissions and longer length of stay. Depression may also have an adverse effect on mortality.

Enquiry about mood change should be a routine part of COPD reviews.

Further reading

Systemic inflammation and co-morbidity

Barnes PJ, Celli BR (2009) Systemic manifestations and comorbidities of COPD. *European Respiratory Journal* **33**; 1165–85

Cote C, Zilberberg MD, Mody SH, et al. (2007) Haemoglobin level and its clinical impact in a cohort of patients with COPD. *European Respiratory Journal* **29**; 923–9

Fabbri LM, Luppi F, Beghe B, et al. (2008) Complex chronic comorbidities of COPD. *European Respiratory Journal* **31**; 204–12

Gan WQ, Man SF, Senthilselvan A, et al. (2004) Association between chronic obstructive pulmonary disease and systemic inflammation; a systematic review and meta-analysis. *Thorax* **59**; 574–80

Hole DJ, Watt GCM, Davey-Smith G, et al. (1996) Impaired lung function and mortality risk in men and women: findings from the Renfrew and Paisley prospective population study. *British Medical Journal* **313**; 711–15

Maurer J, Rebbapragada V, Borson S, et al. (2008) Anxiety and depression in COPD. Current understanding, unanswered questions, and research needs. *Chest* **134**; 43–55 supplement

Sin DD, Wu L, Man SF. (2005) The relationship between reduced lung function and cardiovascular mortality: a population based study and a systemic review of the literature. *Chest* **127**; 1952–9

Sin DD, Anthonisen JB, Soriano JB, et al. (2006) Mortality in COPD; role of comorbidities. *European Respiratory Journal* **28**; 1245–57

Wouters EFM, Celis MPM, Breyer MK, et al. (2007) Co-morbid manifestations in COPD. *Respiratory Medicine COPD Update* **3**; 135–51

4 | Presentation and history

Main points

1 COPD in the UK is uncommon in someone who has never smoked or is a genuinely light smoker.

2 A significant smoking history for COPD is more than 15–20 pack-years.

3 The commonest and most distressing symptom of COPD is breathlessness on exertion.

4 Symptoms are slowly progressive and vary little over periods of weeks.

5 Night-time symptoms are far less common than in asthma, but in severe disease may disturb the sleep of a third of patients. Many patients have more troublesome symptoms in the first part of the morning.

6 A previous history of asthma, atopic illness or childhood 'chestiness' may point to a diagnosis of asthma rather than COPD.

7 Clinical signs of COPD are generally not apparent until the disease is of at least moderate severity.

8 Clinical signs in severe disease include:
   - barrel chest
   - prominent accessory muscles of respiration
   - recession of lower costal margins
   - abdominal breathing
   - weight loss
   - central cyanosis
   - peripheral oedema
   - raised jugular venous pressure

9 Alternative diagnoses must be carefully considered and excluded.

Symptoms

The most common presenting symptoms of COPD are breathlessness on exertion and cough, with or without sputum production. However, considerable loss of lung function can occur before symptoms become apparent, with the result that patients frequently consult their GP only when the disease is at an advanced stage. COPD is a slowly progressive disorder and patients gradually adapt their lives to their disability, not noticing breathlessness until it is severe enough to have a significant impact on their ability to perform everyday tasks. Most smokers expect to cough and be short of breath, and they often dismiss the symptoms of progressive airflow obstruction as a normal consequence of their smoking habit. A smokers' cough, far from being a harmless, insignificant consequence of smoking, is often an early warning sign of COPD.

A recent survey by Partridge and colleagues looked at the frequency of COPD symptoms and the time of day when they most affect patients. Commonly reported symptoms were:

- shortness of breath – 78%

- morning cough with phlegm – 63%

- persistent cough – 60%.

For the person with more severe COPD the time of day distribution for when symptoms are worse were morning 46%, mid-day 11%, afternoon 16%, evening 27% and night 34% (multiple answers were possible). The morning activities most affected were walking up or down stairs, putting on socks/shoes, making the bed, dressing, showering/bathing and drying.

Breathlessness

The most important and common symptom in COPD is 'breathlessness'. This is a subjective term and can be defined as an awareness of increased or inappropriate respiratory effort. Patients describe breathlessness in different ways, but the person with COPD will frequently describe it as difficulty inhaling:

'I just can't get enough air in!'

In health the increased oxygen demand that occurs with exercise is met by using some of the inspiratory reserve volume of the lungs to increase the tidal volume (see Figure 5.11). In COPD, because the calibre of the airways is relatively fixed, the inspiratory reserve volume cannot be fully used. Hyperinflation of the lungs with air-trapping in the alveoli leads to increased residual volume at the expense of inspiratory reserve volume, thus worsening breath-lessness. Dynamic airway collapse due to loss of the 'guy ropes' in emphysema (see Chapter 2) causes further air-trapping, adding to the residual volume and increasing breathlessness on exertion. Flattening of the diaphragms when the lungs are hyperinflated means that the accessory muscles of respiration become increas-ingly important. Any activity, such as carrying shopping or stretching up, that uses these muscles for activities other than breathing will worsen breathlessness. COPD patients often also find it difficult to bend forward, for example to tie shoelaces.

Loss of the alveolar/capillary interface in COPD also means that the increased demand for oxygen that activity imposes cannot be met, and this also increases the sensation of breathlessness.

In asthma, breathlessness is variable; in COPD, it varies little from day to day. The answer to the question 'Do you have good days and bad days?' can thus be illuminating. The other major differences between the breathlessness of COPD and the breathlessness of asthma are that the patient with COPD is rarely woken at night by the symptoms and, until the disease is very severe, is not breathless at rest.

Although breathlessness is slowly progressive, patients will often relate the onset of symptoms to a recent event, notably a chest infection, and will claim to have 'Never been the same since then.' Close questioning will often reveal that the problem is indeed long-standing but that patients have unconsciously adapted their lifestyle to fit the disability. They will perhaps have avoided talking while walking, walked slower than their peers or have started to take the car when they would previously have walked. The chest infection was simply the 'straw that broke the camel's back'.

Cough

A productive cough either precedes or appears simultaneously with the onset of breathlessness in 75% of COPD patients. The cough is usually worse in the mornings but, unlike the asthma patient, the patient with COPD is seldom woken at night. Morning cough and chest tightness are usually quickly relieved by expectoration. Indeed, many patients justify the first cigarette of the day because it helps them to 'clear the tubes'. Morning symptoms in asthma frequently last for several hours.

Sputum

The production of sputum is a common, though not universal, feature of COPD. It is usually white or grey, but may become mucopurulent, green or yellow with exacerbations. It is generally less tenacious and 'tacky' than the sputum in asthma. Excessive production (half a cup full or more) of sputum and frequent infective episodes should raise the possibility of bronchiectasis, and any report of haemoptysis must be taken seriously. You should refer the patient immediately for chest X-ray and a consultant's opinion, because COPD patients have a high incidence of lung cancer.

The production of copious amounts of frothy sputum, particularly if it is associated with orthopnoea or a previous history of hypertension or ischaemic heart disease, may raise suspicions of left ventricular failure and pulmonary oedema.

Wheezing

Wheeze is a common presenting symptom in both COPD and asthma. COPD patients commonly experience wheeze when walking 'into the wind' or going out into cold air. Unlike people with asthma, they are rarely wheezy at rest and are not woken at night by wheeze. The atopic asthmatic will often relate wheezing episodes to exposure to a specific allergen.

History taking

COPD is unusual in a non-smoker, so it is important to quantify an individual's exposure to cigarettes as accurately as possible in terms of 'pack-years'. Smoking 20 cigarettes a day (a pack) for a year equates to one pack-year, 10 a day for a year is one-half pack-year, 40 a day for a year is two pack-years ... and so on. The formula is:

$$\frac{\text{Number smoked per day}}{20} \times \text{Number of years smoked}$$

For example, if a patient smoked 10 cigarettes a day from the age of 14 years to 20 years, that is

$$\frac{10}{20} \times 6 = 3 \text{ pack-years}$$

When doing national service he started smoking seriously! – 20 a day until 45 years of age. That is:

$$\frac{20}{20} \times 25 = 25 \text{ pack-years}$$

Then he made a real effort to cut down and managed to get down to 5 a day until he finally stopped smoking aged 57 years:

$$\frac{5}{20} \times 12 = 3 \text{ pack-years}$$

It is therefore possible to calculate this patient's total cigarette exposure as:

$$3 + 25 + 3 = 31 \text{ pack-years.}$$

A significant smoking history for COPD is more than 15–20 pack-years. If the smoking history is genuinely light, you should look carefully and exhaustively for other causes for the symptoms.

Any exposure to organic dusts, coal dust or welding fumes may be significant, so it is important to find out about a patient's occupational history. Bear in mind, too, that previous jobs might have exposed the patient to agents that could cause persistent, severe, occupational asthma.

It is important to establish when the symptoms started. 'Chestiness' in childhood might have been undiagnosed asthma that has recurred in adult life. Any family history of asthma or a previous history of atopic illness may point to a likelihood of asthma rather than COPD. Smoking predisposes the patient to ischaemic heart disease as well as to COPD, and many older patients will be receiving treatment for hypertension. A full medical history and current drug therapy may highlight the possibility of a cardiac cause for the patient's symptoms.

Excluding other possible causes of breathlessness is very important. (Assessment and differential diagnosis are covered in detail in Chapters 5 and 6.)

Clinical history

A major part of diagnosing COPD is the clinical history. Price and others (2006) have produced a symptom-based questionnaire which helps in finding patients, before performing spirometry to confirm airflow obstruction. Many questions were tested and the seven questions in Table 4.1 were found to provide the most sensitive combination to point to a diagnosis of COPD

Table 4.1 Symptom based questionnaire for identifying COPD in smokers

Question	Response category
Pack years smoked	0–14 , 15–24, 25–49, over 50
BMI	<25.4, 25.4–29.7, >29.7
Does the weather affect your cough??	Yes/no
Do you ever cough up phlegm from your chest when you have a cold?	Yes/no
Do you usually cough up sputum from your chest first thing in the morning?	Yes/no
How frequently do you wheeze?	Occasional or more often/never
Do you have any allergies?	Yes/no

Clinical signs

In mild and moderate disease, clinical signs are mostly absent. It is not until the disease is severe that clinical signs become apparent. *Early COPD is detectable only by measuring lung function with a spirometer.* (Spirometry is discussed in Chapter 5.) More can be gained by inspecting the chest than by examining it with a stethoscope. Removing the patient's shirt and taking a good look can be most informative. Although a definitive diagnosis does not depend on the examination alone, it is still an essential part of the assessment and can be used to support the history and the diagnostic tests. In severe disease the chest may be hyperinflated, with an increased antero-posterior diameter and a typical 'barrel' shape. The ribs become more horizontal and, because the position of the trachea is fixed by the mediastinum, the trachea may look shortened – the distance between the cricoid cartilage and the xiphisternal notch will be less than three finger-breadths. The trachea may also seem to be being pulled downwards with each breath.

Chest percussion may reveal that the liver is displaced downwards by the flattened diaphragms. The usual cardiac dullness on percussion may also be reduced. Relatively quiet vesicular breath sounds may be heard on auscultation. Wheeze may also be audible, as may crackles, particularly at the lung bases. Coarse, fixed crackles may be an indication of bronchiectasis, particularly if the patient is producing larger volumes of sputum.

The strap muscles of the neck may be prominent and the lower intercostal margins drawn in on inhalation (Hoover's sign). Use of the abdominal muscles to aid exhalation may also be apparent, although movements of the rib cage during respiration may be relatively small. The angle between the lower ribs and the sternum – the xiphisternal angle – may widen because the rib cage is raised due to hyperinflation of the lungs. Flattening of the diaphragm may also displace the contents of the abdomen forward, giving the patient a pot-bellied appearance.

In severe disease the effort of walking into the consulting room and undressing will be sufficient to make most patients breathless, and the fact that breathing is hard work will be immediately obvious. They may lean forward, shoulders raised, resting their arms on the table to ease their breathing. Their respiratory rate will be raised and they may use 'pursed-lip' breathing. Their speech may be somewhat 'staccato' because they will not be able to complete a sentence without stopping for breath, and exhalation may be prolonged.

In patients with cor pulmonale the jugular venous pressure (JVP) will be raised, and there will be ankle oedema and central cyanosis. All of these are poor prognostic signs and must be taken seriously. Abnormal blood gases may be associated with loss of mental agility and the ability to concentrate. Elevated carbon dioxide may cause drowsiness and mental confusion, and a typical 'flapping' tremor of the hands when the arms are outstretched.

Finger clubbing is not a feature of COPD but may suggest bronchiectasis or a pulmonary tumour. Weight loss is common in advanced COPD, and another poor prognostic sign. Because malignancy is also a cause of weight loss in this group of middle-aged to elderly smokers, this must be excluded. It is also important to be aware of co-morbidities and to look for anaemia, muscle wasting and signs of cardiovascular disease. Many patients with severe disease will also be anxious and depressed.

Summary

COPD presents as a slowly progressive, non-variable disease that causes breathlessness on exertion and cough with or without the production of sputum. The disease eventually affects every aspect of a patient's life and causes significant disability and handicap. Generally, clinical signs are apparent only when the disease is advanced, and the detection of early disease relies on a high level of suspicion about respiratory symptoms in patients who smoke and the referral of such patients for spirometry.

Further reading

Calverley PMA, Georgopoulos D (1998) Chronic obstructive pulmonary disease: symptoms and signs. In: Postma DS, Siafakis NM (eds) *Management of Chronic Obstructive Pulmonary Disease. European Respiratory Monograph* **3** (May): 6–24

Partridge M, Karlsson N, Small IR (2009) Patient insight into the impact of chronic obstructive pulmonary disease in the morning: an internet survey. *Current Medical Research and Opinion* **25**: 2043–8

Pearson MG, Calverley PMA (1995) Clinical and laboratory assessment. In: Calverley P, Pride N (eds) *Chronic Obstructive Pulmonary Disease*. Chapman and Hall Medical, London; 309–49

Price DB, Tinkleman DG, Halbert RJ, et al. (2006) Symptom – based questionnaire for identifying COPD in smokers. *Respiration* **73**: 285–95

Main points

1 Spirometry measures airflow and lung volumes and is the only accurate method of measuring airflow obstruction in COPD. It is the essential for a confident diagnosis of COPD and for monitoring disease progression.

2 The forced vital capacity (FVC) is the total volume of air that can be exhaled with maximum force, starting from maximum inhalation and continuing to maximum exhalation.

3 The forced expiratory volume in one second (FEV_1) is the amount of air that can be exhaled in the first second of a forced blow from maximum inhalation.

4 Both the FVC and the FEV_1 are expressed as volumes (in litres) and as a percentage of the predicted (reference) value for that individual. Predicted values have been determined from large population studies, and are dependent on age, height, gender and ethnicity.

5 The ratio of FEV_1 to FVC (FEV_1/FVC) is expressed as a percentage or ratio. Values of less than 70% (0.7) are generally considered to indicate airflow obstruction.

6 In diseases that cause airflow obstruction the FEV_1 will be below 80% of the predicted value and the FEV_1/FVC ratio will usually be less than 70%. However, the effect of normal aging on lung elasticity reduces the FEV_1/FVC and a ratio of 0.7 or less may be normal in an asymptomatic elderly person.

7 In severe COPD the FVC may also be less than 80% of the predicted value

8 In restrictive lung diseases both the FEV_1 and the FVC will be below 80% of the predicted value but the FEV_1/FVC ratio will be normal or high.

9 The volume/time trace must be smooth, upward and free of irregularities. The graph must reach a plateau, demonstrating that the patient has blown to FVC.

10 The forced expiratory manoeuvre can also be presented as graphs of flow rate against volume – the flow/volume trace. They show airflow through small airways and can be particularly useful in detecting early airflow obstruction.

11 Pulse oximety should be widely available and routinely measured in primary care settings.

12 Further tests, such as a gas transfer test (TLco) and static lung volumes, are available in lung function laboratories, and may be helpful.

13 Training in the proper use and interpretation of spirometry is essential.

Measuring lung function to determine the presence and severity of airflow obstruction in COPD is as fundamental as measuring blood pressure to detect and monitor hypertension.

Spirometry provides indices not only of airflow, but also of lung volume. The publication of COPD Guidelines since 1997 by the BTS, GOLD, ATS/ERS and NICE, and inclusion of measurement of FEV_1 in the Quality Outcome Framework have encouraged general practices to obtain spirometers. The recently launched consultation document on the National Clinical Strategy for COPD states that the diagnosis should be confirmed by quality assured spirometry.

The widespread availability of primary care spirometry is welcome and brings diagnostic testing closer to patients' homes, but there is concern amongst experts about the quality of recordings and the accuracy of interpretation. Both doctors and practice nurses need training to understand the blowing technique and the interpretation of results.

A recent survey by the British Lung Foundation highlighted some of the difficulties. Of the 750 GPs who responded to the survey more than three-quarters owned or rented a spirometer, but less than a quarter had been trained in obtaining recordings and more than a quarter had had no training in interpreting the results. Equally concerning is a recent survey of practice nurses. Only 20% of the nurses who reported that they used spirometry to diagnose COPD had received accredited spirometry training. A number of studies of primary care spirometry have concluded that the quality of tracings obtained by **untrained** personnel (both nurses and GPs) is poor. Inconsistencies between primary care and specialist reporting of the quality and interpretation of spirometry have also been reported.

Spirometry is a practical skill that needs to be learnt and continually practised if skills are to be maintained. One study has demonstrated a positive correlation between the number of tests performed and their acceptability. Expert opinion is that at least five tests a week (20/month) would be enough to maintain skills, once initial competence had been achieved. Fewer tests than this is unlikely to be sufficient.

'In house' spirometry is one method of providing a spirometry service in a primary care setting, but small practices may be unable to test sufficient patients to maintain the skills of the person doing and interpreting the test, or to make spirometer purchase viable. Suggested alternative models of service provision are:

1   Open access to the local pulmonary function laboratory
2   A PCT-based, peripatetic, expert service
3   A locality based service for a group of small practices.

Where a practice is unable to provide reliable, quality, practice-based spirometry, either because of small numbers of patients or because they lack the expertise, alternative models of service delivery need to be explored.

A document setting out proposed standards for diagnostic spirometry in primary care was published in 2009 (Levy et al. 2009).

Spirometry

What does it mean?

In simple terms, spirometry measures two parameters – **airflow** from fully inflated lungs and the **total volume** of air (the vital capacity) that can be exhaled from maximum inhalation to maximum exhalation. The vital capacity is measured in two ways; as a relaxed and as a forced manoeuvre.

During the forced manoeuvre the patient uses maximum force to blow all the air out as hard and as fast as possible. In a healthy individual this can normally be completed in three to four seconds, but with increasing airflow obstruction it takes longer to push all the air out of the lungs. In severe COPD it may take up to 15 seconds.

The volume of air exhaled is plotted on a graph against the time taken to reach maximum exhalation. Volume is plotted on the x (vertical) axis, and time on the y (horizontal) axis. This is known as the volume/time trace. Three indices can be derived from this trace:

1   FEV_1 – the forced expired volume in the first second.

2   FVC – the total volume of air that can be forcibly exhaled from maximal inhalation to maximal exhalation (the forced vital capacity).

3   FEV_1/FVC – the FEV_1 expressed as a percentage of the FVC (e.g. 76%) or as a ratio (e.g. 0.76).

The FEV_1 and FVC are expressed as absolute values, in litres, and also as a percentage of the predicted value for that individual, depending on their age, height, gender and ethnic origin.

Predicted (reference) values are obtained from population surveys. For example, the predicted (mean) value of FEV_1 for a 30-year-old white male 1.70 metres tall is 3.86 litres and for a 65-year-old woman 1.50 metres tall is 1.7 litres, based on a European Respiratory Society population survey conducted in 1993. Readings 20% either side of this value are considered to be within the normal range. Thus an FEV_1 or FVC over 80% of the predicted value is considered to be normal.

When the airways are normal, 70–85% of the total volume of air in the lungs can be forcibly exhaled in the first second. In other words, the FEV_1 normally comprises 70–85% of the FVC; the ratio of the FEV_1 to the FVC (FEV_1/FVC) is 70–85% (0.7–0.85). This is calculated by dividing the patient's FEV_1 by their FVC and multiplying by 100. When airflow through the airways is obstructed, less air can be exhaled in the first second and the FEV_1/FVC ratio falls. Levels below 70% (0.7) generally indicate airflow obstruction, although this may not be the case in an elderly person. Examples of calculating lung function are given in Table 5.1.

In an effort to simplify the diagnostic criteria for COPD several organisations, including the BTS, NICE and GOLD set a cut-off of

Table 5.1 Calculating lung function in normal and obstructed patterns

Normal	Obstructed
$FEV_1 = 3.0$ litres	$FEV_1 = 1.8$ litres
$FVC = 4.0$ litres	$FVC\ 3.8$ litres
$FEV_1/FVC\% = \dfrac{3.0}{4.0} \times 100$	$FEV_1/FVC\% = \dfrac{1.8}{3.8} \times 100$
$= 75\%$	$= 47\%$

70% (0.7) for FEV_1/FVC. They suggested that levels below this were indicative of airflow obstruction and compatible with a diagnosis of COPD. However, the normal aging process leads to loss of lung elasticity and affects lung volumes. An FEV_1/FVC of 70% may be normal in an asymptomatic elderly person whilst an FEV_1/FVC of 73% may be abnormal in a symptomatic younger person.

There is evidence that the use of a fixed 'cut-off' of 70% of FEV_1/FVC leads to over-diagnosis of airway obstruction in elderly subjects, with the potential for misdiagnosis of COPD and overtreatment, and possible under-diagnosis in younger individuals. The use of the lower limit of normal (LLN) values for FEV_1/FVC minimises this potential. LLN values are based on the normal distribution of results and classify the bottom 5% of the population as abnormal. The ability to produce LLN data is already programmed into spirometer software from major manufacturers.

GOLD, NICE and the ATS/ERS now recognise and acknowledge that use of LLN data is a more reliable method of identifying airflow obstruction, although, for the present all these guidelines have kept the diagnostic 'cut-off' of 70% FEV_1/FVC.

From a practical standpoint it is important to consider a diagnosis of COPD in a younger person whose clinical history and symptoms are compatible with this diagnosis, even if their FEV_1/FVC is greater than 70%. It is also important to consider an alternative diagnosis in an elderly person with an FEV_1/FVC less than 70% whose symptoms are not typical for COPD. In cases of doubt the patient should be referred for specialist opinion and further pulmonary function tests.

The shape of the volume/time trace should be smooth and convex upwards, and achieve a satisfactory plateau indicating that exhalation is complete (Figure 5.1). The FEV_1 is very reproducible and

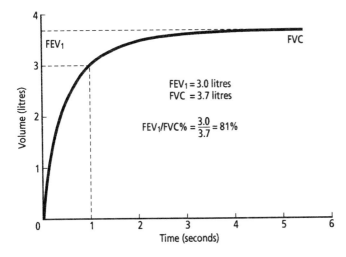

Figure 5.1 Normal Spirometry (volume/time trace)

varies by less than 120ml between blows if the test is carried out correctly. The FVC can show more variation, as it will depend on how hard the subject tries to blow the last remaining air out of the lungs.

The other vital capacity manoeuvre, in addition to the forced expiratory manoeuvre discussed above, is the relaxed or slow vital capacity (VC), in which the patient blows out at their own pace after maximal inhalation. This is a better measure of vital capacity than the FVC, particularly in COPD. When airways are narrowed or unsupported (because of loss of alveolar walls) they tend to collapse during a forced blow, trapping air in the lungs and reducing the volume of FVC. In COPD, the VC is often 0.5 litre greater than the FVC. For this reason it is recommended practice to record a relaxed vital capacity before asking the patient to perform the forced expiratory manoeuvre. If the volume of VC is greater than the FVC the ratio of FEV_1 to VC should be used to determine if airflow obstruction is present, rather than the FEV_1/FVC.

Obstructive pattern

With increasing airflow obstruction it takes longer to exhale and the early slope of the volume/time trace becomes less steep. Figures 5.2 and 5.3 show examples of mild and more severe obstruction.

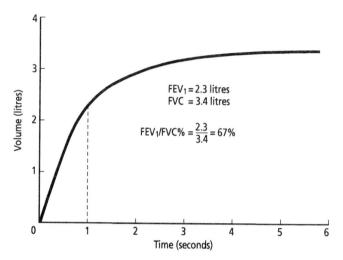

Figure 5.2 Mild obstruction

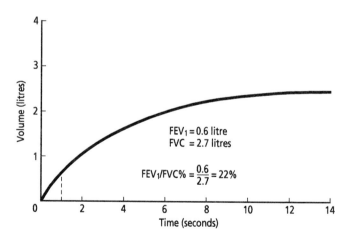

Figure 5.3 Severe obstruction

The FEV_1 is reduced both as a volume and as a percentage of the predicted value and the volume time trace appears 'flattened'. The FEV_1/FVC likewise falls. The FVC in COPD and asthma is usually better maintained at near-normal levels until airflow obstruction is severe.

Restrictive pattern

Spirometry is helpful in the assessment of other respiratory conditions. In patients with, for example, lung scarring, diffuse fibrosis, pleural effusions or rib cage deformity the lung volumes become reduced. Airway size remains normal, which means that air can be blown out at the normal rate. This produces a small but normal-shaped volume/time curve (Figure 5.4) and a normal FEV_1/FVC ratio. The values of FEV_1 and FVC are reduced. This is called a restrictive pattern. Peak expiratory flow (PEF, see below) in such patients is normal. However, a diagnosis of a restrictive lung disease cannot be made on the basis of spirometry alone. If there is clinical evidence for this then the patient should be referred for further pulmonary function tests such as gas transfer and static lung volumes.

Table 5.2 summarises the values for FEV_1, FVC, FEV_1/FVC ratio and PEF in normal, obstructive and restrictive patterns. Table 5.3 categorises the conditions likely to be causing obstructive or restrictive disease.

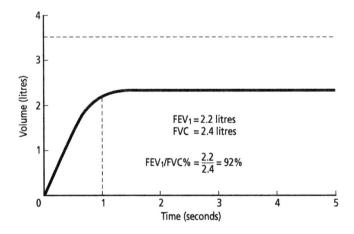

Figure 5.4 Restrictive defect

Table 5.2 Summary of values for FEV₁, FVC, FEV₁/FVC ratio and PEF in normal, obstructive and restrictive patterns

	Normal	*Obstruction*	*Restriction*
FVC	above 80% predicted	above 80% predicted	below 80% predicted
FEV₁	above 80% predicted	below 80% predicted	below 80% predicted
FEV₁/FVC	above 70%	below 70%	above 70%
PEF	above 85% predicted	below 85% predicted	above 85% predicted

Table 5.3 Summary of likely conditions causing obstructive or restrictive disease

Obstructive disease	*Restrictive disease*
Generalised obstruction	Sarcoid
Asthma	Fibrosing alveolitis
COPD	Extrinsic allergic alveolitis
Bronchiectasis	Malignant infiltration
Cystic fibrosis	Asbestosis
Obliterative bronchiolitis	Pleural effusions
	Kyphoscoliosis
Localised obstruction	Ascites
Tumour	Obesity
Inhalation of foreign body	
Post-tracheotomy stenosis	

Blowing technique and reproducibility

Preparing the patient

- The patient should be clinically stable (i.e. at least four weeks should have elapsed since the last exacerbation) and free of respiratory infection.

- For diagnostic spirometry the patient should not have taken a short-acting bronchodilator (beta-2 agonist or anticholinergic) in the last 4–6 hours. Long-acting inhaled beta-2 agonists (including combination products) should be withheld for 12 hours, tiotropium for 24 hours and sustained-release oral bronchodilators (theophyllines and oral beta-2 agonists) for 24 hours.

- The patient should be advised not to eat a large meal within two hours of the test and should avoid vigorous exercise 30 minutes before testing. They should be encouraged to arrive in plenty of time, to rest and relax prior to testing.

- The patient should not be wearing a corset or other restrictive clothing, and should remove any loose-fitting dentures or chewing gum.

- Ensure that the patient is comfortable; invite them to empty their bladder before proceeding.

Some patients find it very hard to do without their short-acting bronchodilators. If they are unable to do without for 4–6 hours, two hours' abstinence is acceptable. Withholding medication is not necessary for routine, monitoring spirometry once a diagnosis has been confirmed. Follow-up tests should be done 'post-bronchodilator' and under the same conditions – at the same time of day and by the same operator – to ensure that results are comparable. Post-bronchodilator FEV_1 is necessary to confirm a diagnosis of COPD and as part of the assessment of its severity.

Blowing technique

The relaxed expiratory manoeuvre should be performed first.

1   The patient should be sitting in an upright position (not standing, because there is a potential risk of their feeling faint or dizzy, especially after repeated blows).

2   Explain and demonstrate the technique to the patient.

3   Put on a nose clip or ask the patient to pinch their nose closed.

4   Instruct the patient to take a maximal breath in through their mouth and then place their lips around the mouthpiece to form an airtight seal.

5   With the minimum of delay between inhalation and exhalation, ask the patient to exhale in a relaxed way (but with some pace – like a big sigh) and to keep exhaling steadily until they cannot exhale any more. You will need to give lots of encouragement to keep exhaling for as long as possible.

6   Allow the patient adequate time – including time for recovery between blows.

Once you have recorded three satisfactory relaxed manoeuvres you can proceed to the forced expiratory manoeuvre. Substitute the instruction below for instruction 5 above:

- With the minimum delay between inhalation and exhalation, ask the patient to exhale as **hard, fast and completely as possible** (with lots of encouragement from you). In a healthy person it may take only 3–4 seconds to complete the blow. With increasing airflow obstruction, it becomes harder to blow air out rapidly and full exhalation can take as long as 15 seconds.

Again, you will need to allow adequate time for the patient to recover between each effort, with a maximum of eight forced manoeuvres in one session.

Technical standards

- A minimum of three technically satisfactory relaxed and forced manoeuvres should be made, giving similar results (good reproducibility) (see Figure 5.5).

- The best two readings of FEV_1, FVC and VC should be within 100ml or 5% of each other, whichever is greater.

Common faults

The most common faults are:

- a slow start to the forced manoeuvre (reducing the volume exhaled in the first second – a falsely low FEV_1 – and an 'S' shape to the beginning of the volume time trace)

- stopping blowing too early (giving a falsely low reading of vital capacity, a falsely high FEV_1/FVC ratio and a volume time trace that fails to plateau)

- coughing during the blow (giving an uneven volume time trace and non-reproducible results)

- submaximal effort (resulting in poorly reproducible results from each blow).

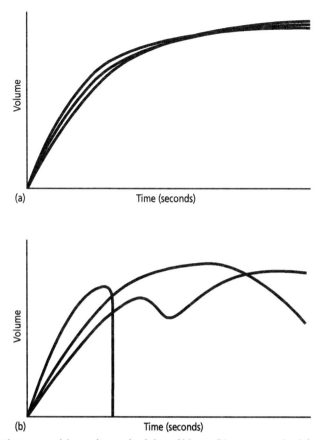

Figure 5.5 (a) Good reproducibility of blows; (b) poor reproducibility

Spirometry is an effort dependent test and the role of the person conducting the test as 'coach' to the patient cannot be over emphasised. It is vital to observe the patient throughout the test and to give maximum encouragement.

Why is FEV₁ the preferred test?

The FEV_1 is the measurement of choice because:

- It is reproducible, with well-defined normal, reference ranges according to age, height, gender and ethnicity.
- It is quick and relatively easy to measure.

- Other diagnostic measurements such as FVC and FEV_1/FVC are recorded, which help in differential diagnosis.

- Variance of repeated measurements in any individual is low.

- FEV_1 predicts future mortality, not only from COPD but also from other respiratory and cardiac disorders.

- FEV_1 is better related to prognosis and disability than FEV_1/FVC; this is mainly because the FVC, depending as it does on effort, is more variable.

The peak expiratory flow (PEF) measures the maximal flow rate that can be maintained over the first 10 milliseconds (ms) of a forced blow. It often under-estimates the degree of airflow obstruction in COPD, and the relationship between PEF and FEV_1 is poor. In milder COPD the PEF may be normal. (In asthma the correlation is better.)

The British, American, European and international COPD guidelines all use a post-bronchodilator FEV_1/FVC of less than 70% (0.7) as indicative of airflow obstruction, and the post-bronchodilator FEV_1 as a percentage of predicted value for estimating the severity of that obstruction. The 2010 NICE Guideline is now in line with GOLD and the ATS/ERS Guidelines. See Table 5.4

Table 5.4 Severity of airflow obstruction

FEV1 % predicted value (post-bronchodilator)	Severity of airflow obstruction		
	ATS/ERS 2004	GOLD 2008	NICE 2010
≥ 80%	Mild	Stage 1 – mild	Stage 1 – mild*
50-79%	Moderate	Stage 2 – moderate	Stage 2 – moderate
30-49%	Severe	Stage 3 – severe	Stage 3 – severe
<30%	Very severe	Stage 4 – very severe**	Stage 4 – very severe**

* Symptoms should be present to diagnose COPD in people with mild airflow obstruction
** or FEV_1 <50% with respiratory failure

Types of spirometer

Spirometers are essentially of two types:

- they measure volume directly (e.g. the dry bellows type of device)
- they measure flow and electronically convert the values into volumes.

Most of the spirometers in use in primary care are electronic flow measuring devices:

- pneumotachographs (Lilly or Fleisch type)
- turbine/rotating vane
- ultrasonic.

These usually have the facility to enter patient's age, height and gender, and will automatically calculate predicted values and the measured values as a percentage of the predicted value. Spirometers from the major manufacturers also have the facility to calculate the LLN.

Spirometers for diagnostic spirometry testing should produce real-time volume time traces of each blow, which can be superimposed on each other, and the variance calculated to assist in assessing reproducibility. Most electronic, flow measuring spirometers also produce a flow/volume curve (see below) as well as the volume/time trace. For diagnostic spirometry the spirometer must also produce a hard copy print out of the results and traces, or have the facility to upload the results and traces to the electronic patient record for inspection. Spirometers that produce number only displays are not suitable for diagnostic spirometry as it is not possible to check the acceptability of the patient's effort.

All spirometers require daily calibration checks with a 1- or 3-litre syringe. This is the only method of ensuring that the machine is recording accurately. A log of calibration checks should be kept for medico-legal reasons. The manufacturers of some electronic devices claim that their instrument is accurate for at least three years and that calibration checks are not necessary between service intervals. This is contrary to international guidelines on spirometry and the national standards document for primary care spirometry. The manufacturer's recommendations for servicing of both the spirometer and the calibration syringe should be adhered to.

Infection transmission from spirometry equipment is extremely rare, but measures to prevent possible cross-infection must be taken. Hand washing before and after handling spirometry equipment is essential and disposable plastic gloves should be worn when handling nose clips and mouthpieces. Nose clips and mouthpieces should be disposable.

It can be difficult to prevent patients accidentally inhaling through the spirometer. For this reason mouthpieces should have one-way valves to reduce this risk. These are a little more expensive than simple cardboard tubes, but they can also be used for peak flow measurement and bulk purchase can reduce costs. Inspiratory manoeuvres are seldom necessary in primary care settings. If these are undertaken then viral and bacterial filters must be used, adding substantially to costs.

Table 5.5 Spirometry training

Basic training	Advanced training
Equipment: • Calibration • Infection prevention and control	Analysis of normal and abnormal spirometry
Patient preparation: • Indications and contraindications • Recording height and weight accurately • Checking and recording patient data	Identifying errors in measurement
Conducting the test: • Instructing the patient and demonstrating technique • Relaxed and forced expiratory manoeuvres • Obtaining maximum effort from the patient	Supervision and quality control of others
Validity and reproducibility: • Recognition of unacceptable results • Techniques for correcting errors	Analysis of the relationship between the spirometry and the patho-physiological changes in the lung
Preparing results for reporting	Advising on subsequent patient management based on the spirometry result.

The spirometer must be cleaned regularly, according to the manufacturer's instructions and a log kept of cleaning procedures. It is also good practice to keep a log of patients tested on the equipment so that, in the event of a patient with infection being inadvertently tested, contact tracing will be easier.

Training in the use of the spirometer and in the interpretation of results is essential. The essential elements of spirometry training are shown in Table 5.5 and should, ideally be subject to assessment. The Association for Respiratory Technology and Physiology (ARTP) and the British Thoracic Society (BTS), have established a nationally recognised qualification assessing competence in both performing and interpreting spirometry in the UK. This is available through the ARTP and other training organisations, where academic accreditation as well as the ARTP/BTS qualification are awarded to successful participants. The ARTP/BTS qualification is the current 'gold standard' for training in the UK. A European Respiratory Society task force is currently developing a spirometry certification programme – a 'European Spirometry Driving Licence'.

Lung age

Some electronic spirometers calculate 'lung age' from the measured and predicted value for FEV_1. If the FEV_1 is reduced, this factor may be used to try to persuade patients to stop smoking – for example, knowing that their lung age is, say, 10–15 years greater than their actual age can be a powerful incentive.

Flow/volume measurement

Most modern spirometers provide a plot of expiratory flow rate throughout the entire expiratory blow at the same time as the standard volume/time trace. A PEF, in contrast, measures only the maximal flow rate that can be sustained for 10 milliseconds and represents flow only from the larger airways. The flow/volume trace, on the other hand, interprets flow from all generations of airways and is more helpful in detecting early narrowing in small airways, as in early COPD. It is also useful for differentiating between asthma and COPD, and can help to determine when there are mixed obstructive and restrictive defects.

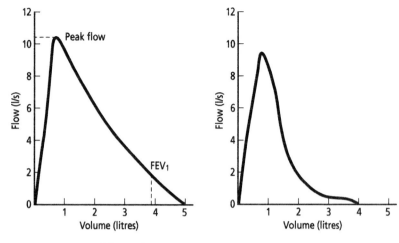

Figure 5.6 Normal flow/volume curve   **Figure 5.7** Mild obstruction

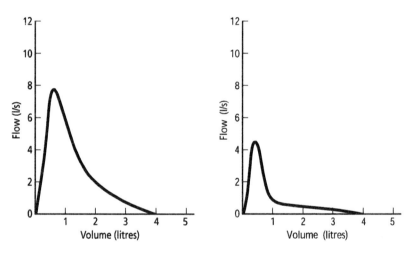

Figure 5.8 Moderate obstruction   **Figure 5.9** 'Steeple' tracing in severe
                                                          emphysema

An understanding of the shape of normal and abnormal flow/
volume curves can be informative and useful. Figures 5.6, 5.7 and
5.8 give examples of normal, mild and moderate airflow obstruction.
Figure 5.9 shows the classic 'steeple' pattern of airway collapse with
emphysema, in which airways suddenly shut down on forced exhalation with low residual flow from the smaller airways. Figure 5.10
demonstrates the restrictive pattern with a normal shape curve and
PEF but small FVC.

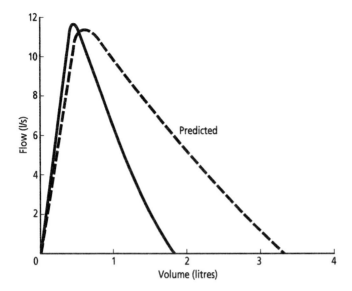

Figure 5.10 Restrictive pattern

Other uses of spirometry

Measuring FEV_1 and FVC provides much more information than a simple PEF. Spirometers can therefore be useful in screening and following a whole range of respiratory disorders and for differentiating between respiratory and non-respiratory causes of symptoms. The main areas of use are:

- obstructive lung disease

- restrictive lung diseases

- diagnosing and monitoring occupational lung disease

- screening of smokers

- medical examinations for scuba diving, aviation and insurance

- health screening and possible screening of new patients (although the value of screening in asymptomatic non-smokers is controversial)

- assessment of patients presenting with undiagnosed cardio-respiratory symptoms, e.g. breathlessness.

Early screening for COPD

In an ideal world, there might be advantages to screening populations at risk – smokers from about 35 years onwards – to detect early indications of airflow obstruction. This could be enhanced with a flow/volume trace, which is the most sensitive, simple test for detecting early changes. In a study from the Netherlands, airflow obstruction was found in 27% of smokers with a cough.

Stopping patients smoking at this stage – admittedly not an easy task – would largely prevent COPD in most of them as well as reducing their risk of lung cancer and cardiovascular disease. There is some encouraging evidence from Poland that patients who are found to have airflow obstruction on general screening are more likely to stop smoking. In the long term there could be considerable cost saving for the nation. NICE have stated that screening for COPD is likely to be cost effective and the National Clinical Strategy strongly supports spirometry for detecting the undiagnosed millions of COPD patients.

Peak expiratory flow (PEF)

PEF is a simple, quick and inexpensive way of measuring airflow obstruction. Its main use is in monitoring asthma.

The PEF meter measures the maximal flow rate that can be maintained over 10 milliseconds and usually detects a narrowing of large and medium-sized airways. It is most effective for monitoring changes in airflow in an individual over time. It has less value diagnostically because, as mentioned earlier, it may under-diagnose the severity of airflow obstruction in COPD.

The blowing technique requires the patient to inhale fully and then make a short maximal blow into the device (a short, sharp 'huff' – likened to blowing out candles on a birthday cake). The reading is expressed in litres per minute (l/min). It should be noted that, because the expiratory blowing technique is quite different from that required for spirometry, the readings for PEF obtained with a flow-measuring spirometer will not be the same as those obtained from a peak flow meter and should not therefore be compared. The result from blowing into a PEF meter is less reproducible than with spirometry, and some patients use some very strange techniques for blowing – from a cough-like action to almost spitting into the device.

PEF can be helpful in COPD but should never be considered diagnostic or quantitative in terms of severity. It may be useful to perform twice-daily readings at home when it is uncertain whether the diagnosis is asthma or COPD.

Pulse oximetry

Approximately 97% of oxygen crossing the alveolar membrane is carried to the tissues attached to haemoglobin, as the unstable compound oxyhaemoglobin. Pulse oximeters non-invasively measure the percentage of available haemoglobin in the peripheral circulation that is saturated with oxygen; the SpO_2 or oxygen saturation. (When oxygen saturation is estimated from an arterial blood gas sample it is termed SaO_2) Oximetry therefore gives a good estimation of how efficiently the lungs are working to get oxygen into the circulation.

The normal range for SpO_2 varies with age. For a young adult of 18–24 years the lower limit is 96.1%. For older individuals, over the age of 64 years the lower limit is 92.7%. For practical purposes a normal range for SpO_2 is 94–98%. Saturations below this should prompt further investigation.

National and international COPD guidelines recommend routine monitoring of oxygen saturation in all patients with moderate and severe COPD in order to detect those patients who are chronically hypoxic and likely to benefit from referral for assessment for long-term oxygen therapy (LTOT). NICE suggest that a saturation of 92% or less in a stable COPD patient indicates the need for referral for LTOT assessment .

Pulse oximeters should be widely available in all health care settings. They can be extremely useful, but also have their limitations. They give no indication of carbon dioxide level and the accuracy of oximetry can be affected by a variety of situations:

- Patients who have cold hands (e.g. due to Raynauds disease or other circulatory problems) will have a sluggish peripheral circulation. SpO_2 will be low

- Accurate oximetry requires a pulsating blood flow. Tremor or cardiac arrythmias can disturb this and lead to inaccurate results

■ Poor positioning of the oximeter probe can also lead to inaccurate results.

Training in the proper use of the equipment is necessary if it is to be reliable and useful.

Gas transfer test (TLco)

This very useful test is performed in hospital lung-function laboratories and relies on the fact that the uptake of carbon monoxide in the lungs is very similar to that of oxygen. The single-breath diffusion test measures the ability of the alveolar air/blood interface to transfer a trace amount of carbon monoxide into the pulmonary circulation. A number of factors affect it, of which the main ones are:

■ the thickness and amount of the alveolar membrane

■ the capillary blood volume

■ the haemoglobin concentration (the test needs to be corrected for haemoglobin level).

Gas transfer is significantly reduced in more severe degrees of emphysema, because of the loss of alveolar tissue. (Gas transfer is also reduced in fibrosing alveolitis, allergic alveolitis and other causes of diffuse fibrosis.) In asthma, gas transfer is normal.

Static lung volumes

Measurement of the total lung capacity (TLC) and residual volume (RV) using a body plethysmograph apparatus is used for assessing patients for lung surgery for COPD and for accurate diagnosis of restrictive lung defects. (See Figure 5.11.)

In emphysema, residual volume is greatly increased, because of the volume of air trapped in enlarged air sacs and by airway collapse due to loss of the 'guy ropes' effect (see Chapter 2).

CT lung scans in inhalation and exhalation can also be used to measure lung volumes.

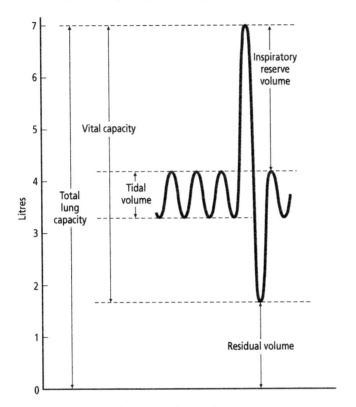

Figure 5.11 Lung volumes

Further reading

Levy M, Quanjer PH, Booker R, et al. (2009) Diagnostic spirometry in primary care: proposed standards for general practice compliant with American Thoracic Society and European Respiratory Society recommendations. *Primary Care Respiratory Journal* **18** (3): 130–47

Booker R (2008) *Vital Lung Function*. Class Health, London

Schermer TRJ, Folgering HTM, Bottema BJAM, et al. (2000) The value of spirometry for primary care: asthma and COPD. *Primary Care Respiratory Journal* **9**: 51–5

6 | Assessment

Main points

1 The diagnosis of COPD is made with a combination of a compatible clinical history of persistent respiratory symptoms, usually a significant smoking history, and confirmation of airflow obstruction with spirometry.

2 All new versions of Guidelines and the Quality Outcomes Framework require diagnostic spirometry to be performed post-bronchodilator. Although formal reversibility testing is not a requirement, in practice performing a baseline reading and then post- bronchodilator spirometry amounts to doing reversibility testing.

3 In cases of diagnostic doubt between COPD and asthma, NICE and the BTS/SIGN asthma Guidelines suggest that an increase in FEV_1 of more than 400ml in response to a bronchodilator or corticosteroid challenge is strongly suggestive of asthma. A smaller response favours COPD but does not exclude asthma.

4 A negative response to a bronchodilator reversibility test does not mean that the patient will not benefit from bronchodilator therapy; therapeutic trials of several weeks' treatment should be undertaken. The response to a bronchodilator reversibility test does not indicate which bronchodilator is likely to give the most symptomatic benefit.

5 Patients with more severe COPD who experience recurrent exacerbations are likely to benefit from long-term inhaled corticosteroids. The response to a corticosteroid reversibility test has no influence on this clinical decision.

6 In patients presenting with severe disease, a referral for arterial blood gases is indicated, especially if the oxygen saturation is less than 92% and there are signs of cyanosis,

raised jugular venous pressure, peripheral oedema or polycythaemia.

7 Other possible causes of the patient's symptoms must be considered and excluded. In the case of continued diagnostic uncertainty, the patient should be referred for a specialist opinion.

8 Formal assessment of disability and handicap should be performed as a baseline from which to assess the effectiveness of any treatment.

9 On review, an assessment should be made of anxiety and depression. There should also be consideration of systemic symptoms of COPD and co-morbidities.

Making the diagnosis and establishing a baseline

Making the correct diagnosis of COPD is based on a combination of a compatible clinical history – persistent respiratory symptoms such as breathlessness, cough and sputum – usually a history of significant smoking, together with confirmation of airflow obstruction on spirometry. The most common differential diagnosis is asthma. Table 6.1 outlines the main differentiating pointers between asthma and COPD.

Table 6.1 The main differentiating points between COPD and asthma

	COPD	Asthma
Current or or ex-smoker	Almost always	Possibly
Symptoms under the age of 35 years	Rarely	Often
Chronic productive cough	Common	Rare – may occur during exacerbations
Breathlessness	Persistent and progressive	Intermittent and variable
Night-time waking with cough and wheeze	Rare	Common
Diurnal or day-to-day variability of symptoms	Uncommon	Common

Patients with late onset asthma, particularly those who have smoked, may pose a difficult diagnostic problem as they often have far less reversibility than young asthmatics. If therapeutic trials are unhelpful, further testing with hospital based tests such as gas transfer factor, and possibly CT scan, may be required.

When the diagnosis is likely to be COPD, a therapeutic trial of bronchodilators can be given and the patient reviewed after several weeks of treatment to assess their response. COPD is unlikely if:

- The FEV_1 and the FEV_1 /FVC ratio return to normal with drug therapy.

- The patient reports a dramatic improvement in their symptoms in response to inhaled bronchodilators.

Performing baseline and post bronchodilator spirometry will help to identify asthmatics.

Bronchodilator reversibility

The main objective of bronchodilator reversibility testing in COPD is to detect patients who have a substantial increase in the FEV_1, and are therefore suffering from asthma.

All updated COPD and asthma Guidelines and the QOF now agree that a significant change in FEV_1 on reversibility testing, suggesting asthma, is more than 400ml. Lesser change is more compatible with COPD. However, not all asthmatics will improve by 400ml and some patients with COPD can increase FEV_1 by over 200ml. Interpretation can thus sometimes be difficult but a good clinical history will often help to clarify the diagnosis.

Reversibility testing was traditionally used to differentiate asthma from COPD and to help determine which bronchodilators were likely to be most effective. However, the evidence-based NICE guidelines have highlighted several problems with this approach:

- There is considerable variation in response from day to day in the same individual, and the results of reversibility tests performed on different occasions can be inconsistent and not reproducible.

- Previously suggested levels of positive response (15% and 200ml improvement in FEV_1) were arbitrary and were not based on evidence.

- Long-term symptomatic response to bronchodilators cannot be determined by the response to a dose of bronchodilator given during a reversibility test.

- Examination of inflammatory cells in bronchial biopsy and induced sputum samples revealed that asthma and COPD could generally be differentiated on the grounds of the clinical history. Reversibility tests were not able to differentiate between the two diseases.

Where diagnostic doubt exists and bronchodilator reversibility tests are being considered, it is important to undertake them when the patient is clinically stable and free of infection.

Small doses of bronchodilator will produce a response in fewer people and therefore high doses of bronchodilator should be used in order not to miss a significant response. The most convenient way to deliver high dose bronchodilators is from a metered dose inhaler (MDI) with a spacer. Alternatives include using a nebuliser. Suitable doses would be 400 μg salbutamol or 80 μg ipratropium, or the two combined.

- Record FEV_1 before and 15 minutes after giving 400 μg salbutamol, or equivalent dose of terbutaline, as four puffs from an MDI via a spacer (one puff at a time). Alternatively record FEV_1 before and 15 minutes after giving 2.5–5 mg nebulised salbutamol, or 5–10 mg nebulised terbutaline.

- Record (preferably on a separate occasion) FEV_1 before and 30 minutes after giving 80 μg ipratropium via a spacer (4 puffs given one at a time) or after giving 500mg nebulised ipratropium.

or

- Record FEV_1 before and 30 minutes after a combination of salbutamol (or terbutaline) and ipratropium.

When the FEV_1 increases by 400 ml or more, this will support a diagnosis of asthma. A response of less than this will support a diagnosis of COPD.

Even when there is no significant reversibility to bronchodilators on formal testing, patients with COPD still benefit from long-
term bronchodilator therapy in terms of improved functional ability
and well-being or decreased breathlessness. Measuring changes in
air trapping in primary care is not possible as you need to measure
Residual Volume. The nearest approximation is to assess a relaxed
vital capacity before and after a bronchodilator – improvements of
400 -600ml can be seen which effectively is the reduction in trapped
air in the lungs. It is thought that bronchodilators of all types have a
major action in reducing air trapping and lung hyper-inflation, thus
improving breathlessness, exercise tolerance and respiratory muscle
mechanics. Trials of several weeks of treatment with different drugs,
different combinations of drugs and different doses are needed to
establish the most effective treatment for each individual. The use of
bronchodilators in COPD is discussed in Chapter 8.

The measures of outcome from therapeutic trials of bronchodilators in COPD are different from those used in the reversibility
testing described above. Improvements in lung function cannot be
anticipated and should not be sought. Improvements in functional
ability and/or breathlessness are more significant. Methods of objectively measuring these rather subjective effects are discussed in
detail later in this chapter.

Measurement of COPD severity

Traditionally the level of $FEV_1\%$ predicted has been used as the main
indicator of disease severity in COPD. Although this is generally
useful and reflects increasing symptoms it has now become apparent
that we need to look at a spectrum of clinical markers and measures of
disability to gain a more complete clinical picture of how the disease is
affecting any given individual. We now better understand that COPD
is a systemic disease which may affect parts of the body other than the
lungs, such as the muscles. Mild airflow obstruction can be associated
with significant disability. A true assessment of severity should therefore not only include spirometry but other measures such as:

- a measure of breathlessness (MRC dyspnoea scale)

- enquiry of how COPD is affecting general daily living

- a CAT (COPD Assessment Test) of quality of life – see page 83

- frequency of exacerbations
- weight loss (BMI)
- oxygen saturation with pulse oximeter
- the presence of cor pulmonale.

UK and International Guidelines previously differed in grading mild, moderate or severe disease based on FEV_1 % predicted. However, the latest NICE update 2010 and the National Strategy have now conformed to the GOLD Guideline severity scale. In Table 6.2 the new (2010) NICE severity levels are on the left of the table and the old levels on the right. NICE has added the stipulation that only patients with respiratory symptoms should be diagnosed with COPD in the Mild stage 1 and not if asymptomatic as their prognosis and change with time is the same as normals. Symptomatic Mild stage 1 patients will need follow up review and treatment if their symptoms are significant.

The prognosis is directly related to the FEV_1 and inversely related to the patient's age. The post-bronchodilator value correlates better with survival than the pre-bronchodilator value:

- Aged under 60   90% 3-year survival
  and FEV_1 above 50% predicted
- Aged over 60   80% 3-year survival
  and FEV_1 above 50% predicted

Table 6.2 Gradation of COPD severity by spirometry – new 2010 update

New NICE clinical guideline severity levels 2010	Post– bronchodilator FEV_1/FVC	FEV_1 % predicted	Old NICE 2004 severity levels
Stage 1 – Mild*	<0.7	>80	
Stage 2 – Moderate	<0.7	50–79	Mild
Stage 3 – Severe	<0.7	30–49	Moderate
Stage 4 – Very severe**	<0.7	<30	Severe

*Symptoms should be present at stage 1 to diagnose patients with COPD with mild obstruction.
** or FEV1 <50% predicted with respiratory failure

- Aged over 60   75% 3-year survival
  and FEV_1 40–49% predicted

A multidimensional assessment of patients has been found to be the best predictor of outcomes such as exacerbations, hospitalisation and mortality. One such is the BODE index which measures BMI, FEV_1 (**O**bstruction), **D**yspnoea on the MRC Dyspnoea scale and **E**xercise with a 6-minute walking test. Inclusion of 6-minute walking test makes this an impractical tool for primary care use, but it is being increasingly used in clinical trials and modified forms, more practical for primary care, may be developed in the future.

Corticosteroid reversibility

A positive response to an oral corticosteroid trial is most likely in patients who have achieved significant reversibility in bronchodilator reversibility tests. Corticosteroid reversibility helps identify people with asthma. It is not a method of identifying which COPD patients need long-term inhaled corticosteroids. As with bronchodilator reversibility tests, corticosteroid reversibility testing should be done during a period of clinical stability.

The NICE guidelines recommend that prednisolone 30mg is given daily for two weeks. The GOLD guidelines suggest that a trial of between six weeks and three months on high-dose inhaled corticosteroids (1000 µg of beclometasone per day or an equivalent dose of an alternative inhaled corticosteroid) may be a safer and more reliable method. Spirometry is recorded before and immediately at the end of the trial. The response should be measured in terms of the *post-bronchodilator* FEV_1. In other words, the FEV_1 is measured after administering an adequate dose of bronchodilator both at the start and at the end of the trial. An improvement of 400ml or more in FEV_1 indicates asthma and patients should be managed according to current asthma guidelines. They are likely to require long-term inhaled corticosteroids.

The usefulness of long-term inhaled corticosteroids in COPD has been the subject of intensive research and their role has become clearer. This is discussed in detail in Chapters 8 and 12.

Other tests to consider in newly diagnosed COPD or in helping to make a diagnosis

- Chest X-ray – should be performed in all new patients, partially to help exclude other causes for their symptoms.

- Full blood count – look for anaemia and polycythaemia. A raised eosinophil count might point to asthma.

- Gas transfer factor – usually normal in asthma but low in COPD. May help to explain patients with mild obstruction who seem disproportionately breathless.

- CT scan – helpful for visualising a range of pathologies and for detecting severity and distribution of emphysema.

- ECG.

- BNP (brain naturetic peptide) and echocardiogram if heart failure is suspected.

Excluding alternative and coexisting pathologies

Lung cancer is an important differential diagnosis to consider. It is 3- 5 times more common in patients with COPD than in non-COPD smokers. Symptoms are often similar, persistent cough being the most common presenting problem. NICE lung cancer guidelines suggest that an urgent chest X-ray should be performed on patients with unexplained or persistent symptoms lasting more than 3 weeks. Over 90% of lung tumours are visible on routine chest X-ray but, if the X-ray is reported as normal and there is still a clinical suspicion of lung cancer, patients should be referred urgently to a chest physician.

It is therefore sound clinical policy to perform a chest X-ray on all newly diagnosed COPD patients. This is to exclude other pathologies rather than to detect abnormal features compatible with COPD. These do not tend to be visible until the disease process is more advanced.

If the chest X-ray reveals 'emphysematous changes' (Figure 6.1) or 'hyperinflation', this will add weight to a diagnosis of COPD, although hyperinflation may also be a feature of chronic asthma. Emphysema may be assessed by computed tomography (CT) – see

Figure 6.2. CT can also be used in the diagnosis of bronchiectasis, a condition found in 29% of COPD patients with persistent cough and sputum as an accompanying disease process.

A chest X-ray may show bullous emphysema, which might be treated surgically. It may reveal cardiac enlargement and pulmonary oedema, prompting cardiac investigation.

The chest X-ray need not be repeated routinely, but an unexplained change in symptoms should be regarded with suspicion. Often the change in symptoms is reported by the patient's carer and

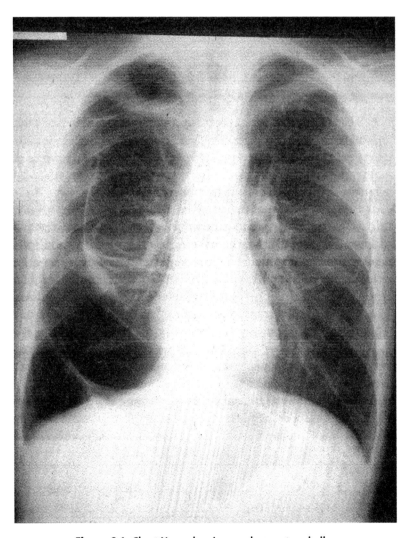

Figure 6.1 Chest X-ray showing emphysematous bullae

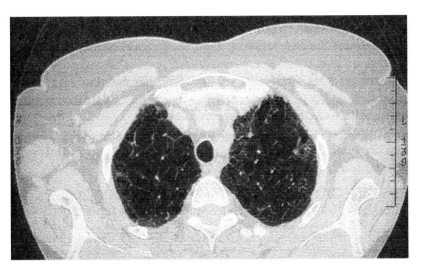

Figure 6.2 A CT scan, showing emphysema

is rather ill-defined and vague: 'He just hasn't been the same recently'. Such a history, failure of a chest infection to resolve or haemoptysis merits a repeat chest X-ray to exclude a tumour.

A review of the patient's current medication may also lend weight to a diagnosis of cardiac breathlessness, or reveal the use of beta-blockade which may have precipitated asthma.

A full blood count should be taken to exclude anaemia, both as a cause of breathlessness and as a co-morbidity. A normochromic anaemia is found in 15% of COPD patients. It may also reveal poly-cythaemia in about 5% of COPD patients – usually those with more severe disease and hypoxia. Oxygen saturation should be measured and referral for arterial blood gases is usually indicated.

The GOLD guidelines recommend referral for arterial blood gases in all patients with an FEV_1 less than 40% predicted. The NICE guidelines recommend referral for patients with severe disease ($FEV_1 <30\%$ predicted) and suggest that referral be considered in patients with less severe disease ($FEV_1 <50\%$ predicted) if they have one or more of:

- cyanosis

- peripheral oedema

- raised jugular venous pressure

- oxygen saturation less than 92%, when clinically stable.

It should be remembered that cyanosis is an unreliable clinical sign and may not become apparent until the oxygen saturation is down to 85% or less. NICE recommends that pulse oximeters should be available in all settings to allow accurate and objective assessment of patients. If the oxygen saturation is over 92%, arterial blood gases may not be necessary at that time.

Oximeters, whilst useful for detecting hypoxia, are unable to detect hypercapnia (raised levels of CO_2). Hypoxia and hypercapnia are common in severe COPD.

Diseases that cause pulmonary fibrosis (e.g. fibrosing alveolitis) may present as breathlessness on exertion and may be confused with COPD. However, the spirometry will not reveal obstruction. The FEV_1/FVC ratio will be normal or high but the lung volumes, the FEV_1 and the FVC will be low. Patients with this pattern of restricted spirometry require assessment by a respiratory physician and are generally beyond the scope of primary care management.

Severe obstructive sleep apnoea (OSA) can present as cor pulmonale. The upper airway obstructs during sleep, producing repeated apnoea sufficient to cause a significant drop in oxygen saturation levels and to rouse the sufferer repeatedly. Patients have a history of 'heroic' snoring and they complain of daytime somnolence. They may have a poor driving accident record because they fall asleep at the wheel. OSA is more common in men than women, and sufferers are often obese, with a collar size of 17 inches or more. Although OSA is an upper respiratory problem and is not related to COPD, it may coexist with it, particularly in patients who are overweight or Cushingoid due to long-term use of oral steroids.

Disability and handicap

Once it has been established that the patient has irreversible airflow obstruction and alternative diagnoses have been excluded, it is important to measure the impact of the disease on the patient's everyday life: the level of disability and handicap. These considerations are frequently overlooked, but it is these effects that are most important to the patient and are the areas that treatment of COPD aims to improve.

Because airways obstruction is largely fixed, big improvements in lung function are not attainable but improvements in disability and handicap are. For the patient such outcomes are far more important than, for example, an improvement of 100ml in the FEV_1, because they equate more with their ability to carry on their everyday lives. You will need a baseline level of disability and handicap from which to assess accurately the effectiveness of any intervention.

The new **CAT (COPD Assessment Test)** (Figure 6.3) is a rigorously developed and validated eight-question, rapid assessment test of symptoms, well-being and activities of daily living. It is derived from the longer, St George's Respiratory Questionnaire and is designed for regular, every day use in primary care. Patients can complete the form at diagnosis and on each visit. The GP or nurse can look at individual questions and the total score to gain insight about clinical, psychological and activity abilities. It should become a routine part of COPD patient assessment.

CAT scores range from 0–40, being divided into four quartiles representing low, medium, high and very high impact on patient

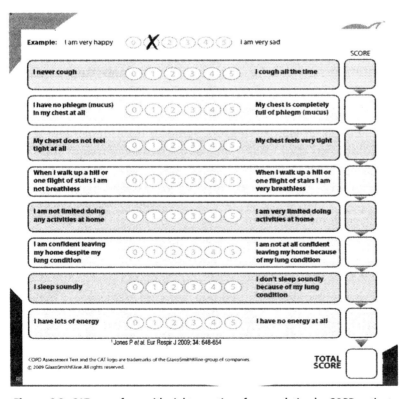

Figure 6.3 CAT score form with eight questions for completion by COPD patients

symptoms and life quality. The clinical markers for CAT scores range from:

- 5 – upper limit of normal
- 10 – impaired quality of life and symptomatic
- 15 – increased risk of death at 1 year
- 20 – increasingly frequent exacerbations.

Somewhat surprisingly a survey of GOLD stage 1 patients gave a CAT score of 16 – medium – which is fairly symptomatic. Stopping smoking can improve the score by 3 points, pulmonary rehabilitation by 2 points, and a single bronchodilator by 1–2 points. Aim for at least 2–5 units improvement in all patients with therapy.

A CAT assessment should be completed every 3 months where appropriate.

Assessing breathlessness

'Breathlessness' is a subjective term, but it is important to quantify this feature because improvement in breathlessness is one of the most important ways of seeing whether treatment is working. There are several scales for assessing it objectively.

The MRC dyspnoea scale (Table 6.3) has been included in the QOF criteria and allows patients to rate their breathlessness according to the activity that induces it. It is graded from 1 to 5 and the results are Read coded. A score of three or more indicates that COPD is impacting on a patient's activities of daily living and should prompt referral for pulmonary rehabilitation and/or a review of medication.

Whilst the MRC scale is helpful and easy to use, it is relatively insensitive to change and may be more valuable as a baseline assessment or monitoring tool rather than a means of measuring the effect of a treatment.

The oxygen cost diagram is more sensitive to change than the MRC scale; it allows the patient to place a mark on a 10cm line, beyond which they become breathless (Figure 6.4). The ability score is the distance in centimetres from the zero point.

Table 6.3 MRC dyspnoea scale

Grade	Degree of breathlessness related to activities
1	Not troubled by breathlessness except on strenuous exercise
2	Short of breath when hurrying or walking up a slight hill
3	Walks slower than contemporaries on the level because of breathlessness, or has to stop for breath when walking at own pace
4	Stops for breath after walking about 100m or after a few minutes on the level
5	Too breathless to leave the house, or breathless when dressing or undressing. Breathless at rest

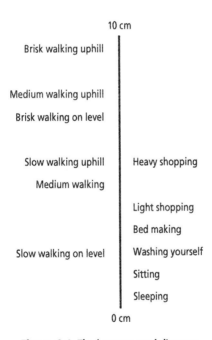

Figure 6.4 The 'oxygen cost' diagram

Other scales allow patients to grade their breathlessness according to the intensity of the sensation. The Borg scale (Table 6.4) is useful for measuring short-term changes in the intensity of the breathlessness during a particular task. It is both sensitive and reproducible.

A simple visual analogue scale is another method of allowing patients to rate the intensity of their breathlessness. As with the oxygen cost diagram, a 10cm line is drawn on a page and the patient

Table 6.4 The Borg scale

0	Nothing at all
0.5	Very, very slight (just noticeable)
1	Very slight
2	Slight (light)
3	Moderate
4	Somewhat severe
5	Severe (heavy)
6	
7	Very severe
8	
9	
10	Very, very severe (almost maximal) Maximal

then marks on the line how intense their breathlessness is, from 0cm (nothing at all) to 10cm (intensely breathless). The score is the distance along the line that the patient has marked.

Assessing walking distance: field tests of disability

A 6-minute walking test and an incremental shuttle walking test are also methods of objectively measuring disability. The six-minute walk measures the distance a patient can walk in six minutes, indoors, on the flat. The patient does a practice walk first, to give them confidence, and measurements are taken on the second walk. The patient is actively encouraged throughout, and stops for rest are allowed. In an incremental shuttle test the patient performs a paced walk between two points 10 metres apart (a shuttle). The pace of the walk is increased at regular intervals, dictated by 'beeps' on a tape recording, until the patient is forced to stop because of breathlessness. The number of completed shuttles is then recorded.

These tests may not be practical for the general practice setting and if neither are feasible you should ask the patient how far they are able to walk; comparisons between walking distance before and after any intervention can still be useful. Asking how many lamp posts the patient can walk past before they get breathless, before and after a given intervention, may be a practical way to assess walking distance objectively in a primary care setting.

If no measurements of walking distance have been taken, the effect of an intervention can be assessed using the CAT test, or by asking:

- Has your treatment made a difference to you?

- Is your breathing easier in any way?

- Can you do some things now that you couldn't do before, or the same things but faster?

- Can you do the same things as before but are now less breathless when you do them?

- Has your sleep improved?

Assessing the impact of the disease on daily activities

The progressively disabling nature of COPD means that it will eventually affect a patient's ability to carry out their normal, everyday activities. The London Chest Activities of Daily Living (LCADL) questionnaire aims to assess this aspect of the impact of COPD. It is a 15-item questionnaire for the patient to complete. It is quick and simple to do. However, it is suitable only for patients with severe disease.

Impact of the disease on psychosocial functioning

Increasing disability and breathlessness on exertion eventually affect all areas of the patient's psychological, sexual and social functioning. An individual's perception of their health status is closely associated with their personality and the amount of social support they have; those with supportive families do better than those who live alone. Some patients with relatively good lung function may be significantly disabled, have given up work and be isolated and depressed, whereas others with appalling lung function may continue to work and remain active and cheerful.

Attacks of breathlessness frequently produce feelings of fear and panic. Episodes in public can cause anxiety and embarrassment, and the wish to avoid such feelings may well sow the seeds of social isolation. Depression is common, particularly in those with severe

COPD. It is a particular problem for those with severe breathlessness and those who are hypoxic. It can significantly affect an individual's ability to cope with the disease and lessen the effectiveness of any therapeutic intervention. Treating coexisting depression can have a very significant beneficial effect on the patient's health status and overall quality of life.

Loss of independence frequently causes feelings of anger, frustration or resentment, often manifested as impatience with the person closest to the patient. Such feelings result in loss of self-esteem and may cause self-destructive behaviour, such as a refusal to stop smoking. The way that patients often cope with these very negative feelings is to withdraw physically and emotionally. Many COPD patients live in an 'emotional straitjacket' (see Chapter 9).

It is important to remain alert to the symptoms of anxiety and depression in COPD patients and screening questions should be asked routinely:

- *'During the past month, have you often been bothered by feeling down, depressed or hopeless?'*

- *'During the past month, have you often been bothered by having little interest or pleasure in doing things?'*

If the answer to either of these questions is 'Yes', then formalised depression screening is indicated.

There are a number of assessment tools that have been used to assess anxiety and depression, though few have been specifically developed and validated for use in COPD. The Hospital Anxiety and Depression Scale (HADS) is frequently used and, despite its name, has been validated for use in primary care settings. It is a self-complete questionnaire, taking up to 5 minutes to complete. A version is available online in the UK, via Mentor. The total anxiety and depression scores are categorised as:

- Normal (0–7)

- Mild (8–10)

- Moderate (11–14)

- Severe (15–21)

A further assessment tool, validated for use in COPD and in patients over 60 years of age is the Brief Assessment Schedule Depression Cards (BASDEC). The Two Question Screen plus Help has also been suggested as a practical method of screening for depression in patients who present with symptoms, or who belong to a high-risk group – such as patients with COPD:

- *'During the past month have you often been bothered by feeling down, depressed or hopeless?'*

- *'During the past month have you often been bothered by little interest or pleasure in doing things?'*

The 'help' question is:

- *'Is this something you would like help with?'*

NICE have published guidelines on the management of depression in adults with long-term medical conditions and these are discussed in more detail in Chapter 10. Standard pharmacotherapy and the 'talking therapies' such as cognitive behavioural therapy, and pulmonary rehabilitation, can have a beneficial impact on depression and anxiety and can improve the patient's quality of life and their ability to cope with the disease. There is, however, some evidence that uptake of pharmacotherapy may be poor, largely due to patient concerns about side effects or misunderstandings of the rationale for it:

'I've got a problem with my lungs not my head!'

It is important to spend time exploring the patient's feelings and explaining the benefits of treatment.

Assessing health status

Assessing health status in COPD, like measuring breathlessness and disability, is important because it too may be improved.

There are several questionnaires available for the measurement of health status, mostly used in hospital rehabilitation programmes and research. The Chronic Respiratory Disease Index Questionnaire is very sensitive to change, but is also the most cumbersome and time consuming to use, and requires training to administer properly.

It was developed as a research tool and is really not practical for everyday use. To overcome some of these problems, a shorter version of this questionnaire, which the patient fills in, has been developed and validated. The St George's Respiratory Questionnaire, a 'self-fill' questionnaire, is more practical and is also available in a shortened version, the AQ20. Another 'self-fill' questionnaire is the Breathing Problems Questionnaire. This is user-friendly and is also available in a short version.

In practice, many of these questionnaires are too cumbersome and time consuming. Their advantages and disadvantages are summarised in Table 6.5. Such formal questionnaires are most useful in the setting of a formal rehabilitation programme. In general practice, a simple enquiry about the two or three most distressing daily activities may suffice. Include questions about the patient's overall feelings of fatigue and about their emotional state. Depression may manifest itself as panic, anxiety or feelings of helplessness and hopelessness.

The degree of control that a patient feels may be assessed by asking such questions as:

- 'How confident do you feel about dealing with your illness?'

- 'Do you feel upset or frightened by your attacks of breathlessness?'

- 'Do you feel in control of your breathlessness?'

- 'Do you feel tired?'

- 'Do you ever feel down?'

Summary

Middle-aged or older patients with respiratory symptoms, particularly those with a significant smoking history, pose a challenge to the health professional. There may have been a tendency to class all breathless smokers as suffering from COPD but it is extremely important not to become blinkered. Asthma can occur at any age, regardless of smoking status. Smokers are at risk of many other smoking-related diseases, such as ischaemic heart disease or lung cancer, and they may have other lung disease or coexisting pathologies that make assessment difficult.

Table 6.5 Health status questionnaires compared

Measure	Description	Advantages	Disadvantages
St George's Respiratory Questionnaire (SGRQ)	76 items Patient self-completes Assesses symptoms, activity, impact on daily life One total score Weighted scoring system	Reproducible and sensitive Well-established and validated in many countries 'Gold standard' measure	Time consuming to complete Complicated to score Some patients have difficulty understanding the questions
AQ20	20 items Patient self-completes Yes/No answers only	Takes 2 minutes to complete and score Repeatable and sensitive	Less sensitive for patients with mild health status impairment
Chronic Respiratory Questionnaire (CRQ)	20 items Both self-fill and interviewer-administered versions Four components (dyspnoea, fatigue, emotional functioning, mastery) Individualised by patient Weighted scoring system	Reproducible and sensitive Well studied	Time consuming to complete and score Scoring system complicated

It is therefore extremely important that history taking is thorough and comprehensive and that alternative diagnosis is ruled out. It is also vital that patients are reviewed to assess their response to treatment and, when there is any degree of diagnostic uncertainty, further tests carried out to confirm or refute a diagnosis of COPD. Failure to assess patients properly may lead to misdiagnosis and inappropriate treatment. All patients deserve a thorough assessment to make sure that other pathologies are not missed and that appropriate treatment is given and its effectiveness properly assessed.

Further reading

Assessment of impairment

Burrows B (1991) Predictors of cause and prognosis of obstructive lung disease. *European Respiratory Review* **1**: 340–5

Callahan CM, Cittus RS, Katz BP (1991) Oral corticosteroid therapy for patients with stable chronic obstructive pulmonary disease: a meta-analysis. *Annals of Internal Medicine* **114**: 216–23

Roberts CM, Bugler JR, Melchor R, et al. (1993) Value of pulse oximetry for long-term oxygen requirement. *European Respiratory Journal* **6**: 559–62

Assessment of disability

Borg G (1982) Psychophysical basis of perceived exertion. *Medicine and Science in Sports and Exercise* **14**: 377–81

Garrod R, Bestall JC, Paul EA, et al. (2000) Development and validation of a standardized measure of activity of daily living in patients with severe COPD: the London Chest Activity of Daily Living Scale (LCADL). *Respiratory Medicine* **94**: 589–96

McGavin CR, Artvinli M, Naoe H (1978) Dyspnoea, disability and distance walked: a comparison of estimates of exercise performance in respiratory disease. *British Medical Journal* **2**: 241–3

Noseda A, Carpeiaux JP, Schmerber J (1992) Dyspnoea assessed by visual analogue scale in patients with obstructive lung disease during progressive and high intensity exercise. *Thorax* **47**: 363–8

Singh SJ, Morgan MDL, Scott SC, et al. (1992) The development of the shuttle walking test of disability in patients with chronic airways obstruction. *Thorax* **47**: 1019–24

Williams SJ, Bury MR (1989) Impairment, disability and handicap in chronic respiratory illness. *Social Science and Medicine* **29** (5): 609–16

The BODE index

Celli RB, Cote CG, Marin JM, et al. (2004) The Body Mass Index, airflow obstruction, dyspnea, and exercise capacity index in chronic obstructive pulmonary disease. *New England Journal of Medicine* **350**; 1005–12

Assessment of handicap

Dudley DL, Glaser EM, Jorgenson BN, et al. (1980) Psychosocial concomitants to rehabilitation in chronic obstructive pulmonary disease. *Chest* **77** (3): 413–20

Guyatt GH, Berman LB, Townsend M, et al. (1987) A measure of quality of life for clinical trials in chronic lung disease. *Thorax* **42**: 773–8

Hyland ME, Bott J, Sing S, Kenyon CAP (1994) Domains, constructs and the development of the breathing problems questionnaire. *Quality of Life Research* **3**: 245–56

Jones PW, Quirk FH, Baveystock CM, et al. (1992) A self-complete measure for chronic airflow limitation: the St George's questionnaire. *American Review of Respiratory Disease* **147**: 832–8

Jones P, Harding G, Wiklund I, et al. (2009) Improving the process and outcome of care in COPD: development of a standardised assessment tool. *Primary Care Respiratory Journal* **18** (3); 208–15

O'Brien C, Guest PJ, Hill SL, Stockley RA (2000) Physiological and radiological characterisation of patients diagnosed with chronic obstructive pulmonary disease in primary care. *Thorax* **55**: 635–42

Addresses for questionnaires

COPD Assessment Test (CAT)
Available on line at: www.catestonline.org

Chronic Respiratory Disease Index Questionnaires
Peggy Austin and Dr Holger Schünemann
Room 2C12
McMaster University Health Sciences Centre
Hamilton, Ontario L8N 3Z5
CANADA
Email: austinp@mcmaster.ca or schuneh@mcmaster.ca

St George's Respiratory Questionnaire
Professor Paul Jones
Division of Physiological Medicine
St George's Hospital Medical School
Cranmer Terrace
London SW17 0RE

Breathing Problems Questionnaire
Professor Michael Hyland
Department of Psychology
University of Plymouth
Plymouth
Devon PL4 8AA

London Chest Activities of Daily Living
Rachel Garrod, PhD, MSc, MCSP
School of Physiotherapy,
St George's Hospital Medical School,
Cranmer Terrace
Tooting,
London SW17 0RE

Smoking cessation

Main points

1 Stopping smoking is the only intervention that significantly affects the natural history of COPD.

2 The smoking status of all patients should be recorded and smokers reminded, at every suitable opportunity, of the benefits of quitting. Recording smoking status and giving smoking cessation advice is rewarded under QOF.

3 Brief advice can be effective in persuading people to stop smoking. All healthcare professionals should be trained in giving brief smoking cessation advice and be able to refer smokers who want to stop to their local NHS Stop Smoking Service.

4 NICE have published guidance on Smoking Cessation Services and the use of pharmacological aids to smoking cessation – nicotine replacement therapy (NRT), buproprion and varenicline. These can significantly increase long-term quit rates and their appropriate use should be encouraged.

5 The choice of pharmacological aid should be made in consultation with the patient and take account of their personal preferences as well as any contraindications and potential for adverse effects.

6 Advice, support and encouragement, including a referral to Smoking Cessation Services should be offered to all smokers attempting to quit. Support, particularly through the critical first few weeks of a quit attempt, can increase their chances of success.

7 NRT can be offered to smokers who do not want to stop abruptly, but wish to reduce their smoking as a prelude to stopping, as part of the nicotine assisted reduction to stop (NARS) strategy – also known as 'cut down to quit', or 'cut down to stop'.

8   Smokers who show a high level of dependence may be offered a combination of NRT patches and another form of NRT, such as gum, inhalator, lozenge or nasal spray.

Stopping smoking is the single most important intervention in COPD and the only thing that significantly alters the natural history of the disease. It is of primary importance at every stage and must be encouraged actively and continuously. In mild COPD it may be the only treatment needed and may prevent the patient ever developing severe, disabling and life-threatening illness.

Unfortunately, persuading patients to stop smoking is often difficult, and failure can be demoralising and disheartening for patient and health professional alike. Most ex-smokers have made several serious attempts to stop before they eventually succeed.

Nationally the prevalence of smoking in people over the age of 16 years is 21%. Smoking rates have fallen dramatically since the 1970s, particularly in the higher socio-economic groups. However, smoking rates remain highest among lower socio-economic groups and are the primary cause of the gap in life expectancy between rich and poor. In men, smoking is responsible for more than half the excess risk of premature death between the social classes. Rising tobacco taxation and increasing evidence of the harmful effects of smoking have little effect on people in these groups. Perversely, those who can least afford it – the economically deprived – are those who tend to smoke, continue to smoke and smoke most!

On the positive side, the introduction of the ban on smoking in public places and places of work has helped to reduce smoking prevalence rates and is set to save a large number of lives. Since the publication of *Smoking Kills* in 1998 there has been a concerted and vigorous campaign by the UK Department of Health, supported by smoke free legislation, to reduce smoking. Health education messages about the long-term effects of smoking, together with pharmacological aids to smoking cessation on prescription, accessible NHS Smoking Cessation Services and the encouragement under QOF for primary care to adopt a systematic approach to smoking, seem to be having an effect. From 1998 to 2008 2.5 million people have successfully quit the habit.

Why do people smoke?

The reasons why people start smoking and continue to smoke in the face of mounting evidence of its harmful effects are complex.

Most smokers start in adolescence, when it may be seen as a 'rite of passage' to adulthood. There may be considerable and irresistible peer group pressure to smoke. Smoking may be one of those 'risk-taking' or rebellious behaviours that are a normal part of growing up. Unfortunately, a third of the adolescents who start will become life-long smokers. Between 1998 and 2002, in England alone, smoking caused an annual average of 86,500 deaths; around 240 adults die of a smoking-related disease every day. The tobacco industry needs to recruit new smokers to replace them.

Restrictions on advertising and the raising of the legal age for buying cigarettes from 16 to 18 years in 2007 have reduced smoking rates in the 16–18 year age group from 24% to 17% between October 2007 and June 2010. Unfortunately there has been no effect on smoking prevalence in the over 18s. However, around 80% of smokers start before the age of 19 years, so the trend is encouraging.

Nicotine is highly addictive and, once 'hooked', smokers are adept at adjusting their smoking to satisfy their need for nicotine without taking in so much that they suffer side-effects. Nicotine is a powerful neural stimulant, acting on the pleasure centres of the brain. Stimulation is followed by rebound depression and the addicted smoker then feels the need for another cigarette. The biochemistry of a nicotine-addicted brain is different from that in a 'normal' brain.

- The cigarette is a highly efficient nicotine-delivery system. Nicotine is absorbed very rapidly across the lungs and reaches the brain quicker than if it were injected intravenously.

- If the number of cigarettes smoked a day is reduced, the smoker will take longer and deeper puffs to get the same amount of nicotine.

- Simply reducing the number smoked or switching to a lower tar cigarette is seldom successful as a quitting strategy, although reducing the number smoked in combination with NRT (the NARS strategy) may increase the likelihood of an eventual quit.

- Cigarette smokers who switch to cigars are likely to inhale the cigar smoke and get an even higher tar load into the lungs than with cigarettes.

Nicotine, although addictive, is a relatively harmless drug. It is the other constituents of tobacco that cause damage. Cigarette smoke contains upwards of 4000 different chemicals, 600 of which are known carcinogens. Perrier water was withdrawn from sale when it was found to contain 4.7g per litre of benzene, a known carcinogen. A single cigarette delivers 190g of benzene.

Addiction to nicotine is the main reason why smokers find it hard to stop, but there are other factors. Each cigarette is 'puffed' about 10–12 times, and 20 cigarettes a day is associated with 200–250 hand-to-mouth movements every day: 91,250 movements a year. A powerful habit. Smoking becomes associated with pleasurable everyday activities: having a cup of coffee, relaxing after a meal, watching the television, etc. It may be associated with pleasurable memories and social activities. When smokers try to quit they not only have to cope with withdrawal of an addictive drug but also with the loss of an 'old friend' that might have been part of their lives for many years. Fear of failure may be another powerful reason why a smoker does not make any move to stop. Physical addiction and habit together serve to make smoking a very difficult habit to break.

How can smokers stop smoking?

In order to stop, the smoker has to *want* to stop. This sounds pain-fully obvious but the path from 'contented smoker' to serious 'quitter' is tortuous and one where advice from you can have a consider-able influence. Some health professionals find it difficult to engage with smokers about their behaviour, fearing that advice to give up may damage their relationship with that patient and 'scare them off'. Raising the subject needs to done sensitively and in a non-threatening manner. The use of 'open' questions that encourage the smoker to talk about their habit and how they feel about stopping can be a helpful way of beginning to address the issue. Nearly 70% of smokers, when asked, say they would like to stop, so constructive advice, support and encouragement might help them to move from a period of contemplation to doing something serious about quitting. Tagging the medical records and bringing up the subject of smoking in a non-threatening way at every attendance can be highly effective and may prompt a 'contented smoker' to contemplate stopping, or a smoker who is contemplating stopping to making a serious attempt to stop. Showing concern, acknowledging the difficulties of quitting and offering practical advice and support are perhaps most helpful. A censorious approach is likely to produce only resistance, and a lecture about the harmful effects of smoking is likely to be counter-productive. Smokers know that their habit is harmful! It is more effective to ask what they think would be the benefits of stopping and to relate and reinforce those benefits in relation to their own health. For a smoker with COPD this is relatively easy. Relating their own lung function to what it would be in a healthy non-smoker (see Figure 2.1) could be a powerful incentive to take a serious step to becoming an ex-smoker. Positive encouragement that stopping smoking is a really effective and important step that they can take to help themselves, together with reassurance that you will be there to help, may be the best approach.

A dramatic event (e.g. a myocardial infarction) that makes a patient anxious about their health is often a trigger to action. Unfortunately, slowly progressive breathlessness seldom produces the same trigger, but a recent unpleasant chest infection or exacerbation of COPD might. Targeting patients when they are most susceptible to advice may increase success rates.

What kind of support works?

Publicly funded, NHS Stop Smoking Services are available throughout the country and have helped large numbers of smokers to successfully stop. NICE issued public health guidance on smoking cessation services in 2008, highlighting a number of smoking cessation activities proven to be effective.

Brief interventions

This typically takes less than 10 minutes and should be delivered by all healthcare professionals – doctors, nurses, pharmacists, etc. The exact content of a brief intervention package will depend on the smoker's receptiveness to advice and their willingness to consider stopping. It may include:

- Opportunistic advice

- An assessment of their readiness and commitment to a quit attempt – 'Have you every tried to stop?' followed by 'Are you interested in stopping now?'

- Pharmacotherapy and/or behavioural support

- Self-help material

- Referral to a Stop Smoking Service for more intensive support.

Individual behavioural counselling

The smoker has face-to-face meetings with a counsellor trained in smoking cessation. These are typically scheduled weekly, over a period of at least 4 weeks after the quite date. This is normally combined with pharmacotherapy.

Group behaviour therapy

Again, this is normally combined with pharmacotherapy. Meetings take place weekly for the first 4 weeks of a quit attempt and the group receives information, advice and some form of counselling, such as cognitive behavioural therapy, from a trained counsellor.

People who are referred to a Smoking Cessation Service are more likely to quit than those who 'go it alone', but not all individuals are prepared to join a group or wish to go to a specialist service. The NICE guidance on the use of pharmacotherapy for smoking cessation states that smokers should be offered '… advice, encouragement and support **or** a referral to a smoking cessation service.' Counselling is a key factor for success in smoking cessation and the policy in most areas is for smokers to be referred for this, either to a trained individual at the GP surgery or to the local Smoking Cessation Service, before prescribing pharmacotherapy on the NHS. GPs may still prescribe, after giving advice, when a smoker is first seen, but the advice and support is still recommended.

Once a patient has decided to make a serious attempt to stop smoking, practical advice on how to cope and support through the first critical three months of stopping are most beneficial – in whatever setting this takes place. Self-help materials and telephone helplines are additional means of supporting smokers through the quit process.

Follow-up appointments at one week, three weeks, two months and three months after stopping to offer support and encouragement may be helpful. If resources in primary care are strained, the most important period to concentrate on is the first month. It may take several serious attempts before a smoker makes the final transition to ex-smoker. In the event of relapse, it is important not to condemn but rather to support and encourage the patient to try to identify why they have failed, develop a strategy for avoiding failure in the future and to make another serious attempt. As Mark Twain famously remarked:

'Stopping smoking is easy. I've done it hundreds of times.'

Pharmacotherapy

For some smokers, withdrawal symptoms such as irritability, nervousness and cravings may cause relapse and unwillingness to make another attempt to quit. The pharmacological aids to smoking cessation – NRT, buproprion and varenicline can at least double a smoker's chance of long-term smoking cessation. Quit rates are maximised when these therapies are combined with some form of behavioural support and all smokers prescribed these aids should be strongly encouraged to attend.

NICE recommends that pharmacotherapy should only be given if a smoker is ready to set a 'quit date' and that any prescription should only be sufficient to last for 2 weeks after that date – normally 2 weeks of NRT or 3-4 weeks of buproprion or varenicline. Repeat prescriptions should then only be issued if the individual has demonstrated that they are really attempting to stop. These restrictions allow for re-assessment and continuing support, and will help ensure cost-effective prescribing.

Nicotine replacement therapy

Nicotine replacement therapy (NRT) can be very effective; large, placebo-controlled trials have shown that it can approximately double quit rates at one year. It is available in six forms:

- chewing gum
- transdermal patch

- inhalator
- nasal spray
- sublingual tablet
- lozenge.

Figure 7.1 shows the different blood nicotine levels with the different types. All forms of NRT are available both 'over the counter' at pharmacists and on prescription in the UK.

Nicotine gum: is the oldest form of NRT and is available in two strengths (2mg and 4mg) and a variety of flavours. The gum should be chewed until it starts to produce a flavour and then 'parked' between the cheek and the gum. If it is chewed continuously, it tastes unpleasant. When the desire to smoke is felt again, the gum is chewed and parked again. Each piece of gum lasts about 20 minutes and up to 16 pieces can be chewed in 24 hours. Nicotine is absorbed from the lining of the mouth, the buccal mucosa, and produces a peak in venous nicotine levels similar in shape but less than that achieved by smoking. It is suitable for the highly addicted smoker because it is used on demand.

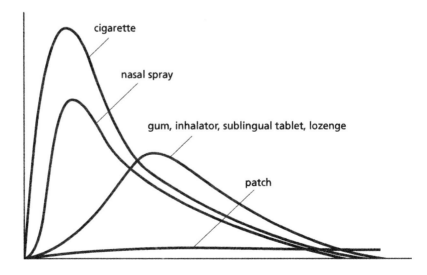

Figure 7.1 Blood nicotine levels with different types of nicotine replacement therapy

Nasal spray: can produce peaks in nicotine level higher than those obtained with the gum but still considerably lower than those achieved with cigarettes. The nicotine is absorbed from the nasal mucosa. It should not be sniffed up the nose but sprayed onto the mucosa when the desire to smoke is felt. Up to 64 'puffs' a day can be used. This form of NRT most closely resembles the effects of smoking and is most suitable for the very heavily addicted smoker.

Nicotine inhalator: produces peaks in nicotine levels similar to those from nicotine gum. The inhalator contains a mentholated plug impregnated with nicotine, and is sucked when the desire to smoke is felt and until that desire goes away. Nicotine is absorbed from the buccal mucosa. Each plug lasts for about 20 minutes.

Transdermal nicotine patches: are easy to use. They are of two types (16 hour or 24 hour), and come in several strengths. Patches do not produce peaks in nicotine levels to mimic the effect of smoking but, rather, provide a steady background level. The rationale behind the 24-hour patch is to prevent the strong urge to smoke that many smokers feel first thing in the morning, caused by an overnight fall in nicotine levels. They may, however, produce sleep disturbance or nightmares, and the adhesive in the patches can cause local skin irritation.

Sublingual tablets: are dissolved under the tongue when the desire to smoke is felt. The peak in nicotine level obtained is similar to that achieved with gum or the inhalator, and, because they too are used on demand, sublingual tablets are suitable for heavily addicted smokers. Unlike the other forms of NRT, these tablets are licensed for use during pregnancy, if the woman is unable to stop smoking without using NRT.

Lozenges: are also used on demand and are suitable for the heavily addicted smoker. They produce peaks in nicotine levels similar to those achieved with sublingual tablets, inhalator and gum. One or two lozenges can be sucked per hour, when the urge to smoke is felt.

The principle of NRT is to replace the nicotine a smoker takes in, although at considerably lower levels, thus reducing withdrawal symptoms and allowing the smoker to concentrate on changing the habits of smoking. When the habit is broken, the amount of nicotine can be reduced over a period and the NRT withdrawn. It is important that the smoker understands at the outset that it is not intended to replace cigarettes and will not be a substitute for will power. A considerable amount of nicotine will be given up from day one. In order for NRT to work, the smoker has to be motivated to stop! It is not suitable for the genuinely light or social smoker, because it may provide more nicotine than they are accustomed to and produce toxic side-effects.

To maximise success with NRT it may help if you match the smoker to the product and ensure that the smoker's expectations of the effects of NRT are realistic. Instruction in how to chew the gum or use the inhalator may prevent problems with incorrect use. Failure with NRT is often due to:

- stopping therapy too soon

- not using high enough doses because of fears about side-effects.

The list of possible side-effects on the side of a packet of NRT can be daunting. Fear of side-effects may also be used as an excuse not to attempt to stop smoking, and some smokers are concerned about becoming addicted to the NRT. This is in fact a rare occurrence, so you can reassure patients that this is unlikely.

It is important that patients understand that the side-effects of NRT are the same as the side-effects of smoking but that the risks of using it are considerably less than those of continuing to smoke. Except for the sublingual tablets (see earlier) NRT is not licensed for use by pregnant or breast-feeding women because of the lack of research into its teratogenicity. However, The British National Formulary suggests that intermittent therapy with oral NRT preparations, patches that are removed at night, or a combination of the two, can be used in both situations if non-pharmacological methods are failing. Careful, clinical judgement needs to be exercised. It is also advised that NRT not be used:

- within three months of a myocardial infarction

- within three months of a cerebrovascular accident

- by people with active peptic ulceration

although for these patients the risks of continuing to smoke are probably considerably higher.

Transdermal patches should not be used by patients with extensive skin disease; the other types of NRT – chewing gum, nasal spray, inhalator, sublingual tablets or lozenges – should be used instead.

Generally, NRT should be taken for 12 weeks with a two- to four-week period at the end of the course when the dose is reduced. The benefits of using NRT and stopping smoking massively outweigh the risks of continuing to smoke, and helping patients to come to grips with the reality of the risks may be helpful.

Two different forms of NRT – patches and gum, for example – may be prescribed concurrently if the smoker is very heavily dependent and unable to stop. However, specialist care may be advisable for such 'problem' smokers.

Nicotine assisted reduction to stop (NARS)

Prior to September 2005 the licence for all forms of NRT stipulated that smokers should stop smoking completely when starting NRT therapy. Although 70% of smokers say they want to quit only 12% are ready to stop in the next month, making only a small percentage suitable for an abrupt cessation strategy. The MHRA have now approved a new application for the use of the NRT inhaler and gum, allowing for longer term use in people who do not want to stop smoking abruptly, but want to use NRT to help them cut down their cigarette consumption. That complete cessation is the ideal must always be stressed, but a reduction in consumption – 'harm reduction', although not a substitute for stopping – is a step in the right direction. The evidence now suggests that smokers who achieve a sustained reduction using NRT are more likely to eventually stop completely, even if this was not their original intention.

The process for a 'cut down to quit' using NRT is:

- 0–6 weeks – cut down to 50% of baseline consumption (this should be confirmed by at least a 1 part per million drop in exhaled carbon monoxide)

- 6 weeks–6 months – continue to cut down and stop completely by 6 months

- 6–9 months – stop smoking completely and continue using NRT

- Within 12 months – stop using NRT.

A recent systematic review of seven NARS trials, using NRT for between 6 and 18 months, has demonstrated twice the sustained quit rate for smokers using NRT compared with placebo. There were no significant adverse effects from taking NRT for this prolonged period. The smokers recruited for these trials had either no intention of stopping completely, or were unable to attempt an abrupt quit. However, these trials also combined NRT with behavioural support, so it remains unclear whether NARS without support would be as effective.

The current NICE guidance states that smokers wishing to use a NARS approach to stopping smoking can be given the appropriate support and prescribed NRT on the NHS, but only if it is part of a properly controlled research study. NRT advertising to the general public, however, contains information about its use for 'cut down to quit', so there are bound to be smokers buying NRT over the counter using a NARS strategy, with or without support, in an uncontrolled way.

Bupropion

Bupropion was initially developed as an antidepressant. It works directly on the addiction pathways in the brain and helps to prevent cravings for nicotine rather than replacing one nicotine delivery system with another. It can be very effective, although, like NRT, it is not a replacement for will power and the smoker has to be motivated to stop. Several large, placebo-controlled studies have demonstrated its effectiveness and it has been endorsed by NICE as a cost-effective therapy.

An agreed 'quit date' is set at about 10–17 days into the course of treatment and the smoker can continue to smoke until then. One bupropion 150mg tablet a day is taken for six days then one twice daily, at least eight hours apart, for the remainder of the two-month course. The smoker stops smoking on the quit date but continues taking bupropion for a full eight weeks. The tablets can then be stopped abruptly. If the smoker has failed to stop after one month of treatment, they are unlikely to succeed and consideration should be given to stopping treatment after one month.

Bupropion is generally well tolerated. Side-effects such as insomnia, dry mouth, nausea, agitation or a generalised rash are experienced by a few smokers but these are usually mild and usually disappear once treatment is stopped.

There are some contraindications to its use, and prescribers and those who advise smokers must be fully conversant with them. They are:

- current or past seizures

- current or past eating disorder (e.g. bulimia or anorexia nervosa)

- history of bipolar disorder (e.g. manic-depressive psychosis)

- severe hepatic cirrhosis

- brain tumour

- undergoing withdrawal from alcohol or benzodiazepines.

The prescribing information for bupropion also counsels caution when using this drug in smokers with any predisposing risk factors for seizure, such as concurrent use of other antidepressants, antipsychotics or theophyllines. Careful enquiry should therefore be made about concurrent drug use – including over-the-counter therapies such as St John's wort – and previous medical history.

When bupropion was first introduced in the UK there were a few, highly publicised, deaths associated with its use. However, that there was a causal link between the use of bupropion and these deaths was not proven. Most of the patients who died had underlying smoking-related conditions and some were not taking the drug at the time of their death. Others had contraindications to the use of bupropion that had not been reported to the prescriber.

Varenicline

Varenicline, a nicotine receptor partial agonist, is the newest addition to the pharmacological aids to smoking cessation and some studies have demonstrated superior effectiveness over both NRT and bupropion. It has a dual action – partially stimulating the nicotine receptor without producing the full effect of nicotine on the brain's pleasure centres, and simultaneously blocking the ability of nicotine to bind to the receptor. It can therefore both reduce cravings for cigarettes and decrease their pleasurable effects.

Varenicline is available as 0.5 mg and 1 mg tablets. The smoker sets a 'quit date' 10–14 days into the course of treatment. A 0.5mg tablet is taken once daily for the first three days of treatment. From days four to seven the dose is increased to 0.5mg twice daily. From day eight a 1g tablet is taken twice daily to the end of the 12-week course. NICE have approved its use for only 12 weeks but it can be extended to 24 weeks in quitters who still have strong withdrawal symptoms. Studies indicate that sustained quit rates may be substantially improved by taking varenicline for 24 weeks.

Nausea and other gastrointestinal side effects, such as vomiting may occur. It may also cause dizziness or sleepiness and patients should be warned not to drive or operate heavy machinery until they know how they will be affected. Varenicline is excreted through the kidney and care should be exercised in prescribing to patients with reduced renal function. It should not be given to pregnant or breast feeding mothers.

In 2009 the US Food and Drug Administration required varenicline to carry a 'black box' warning – their strongest safety warning – due to concerns from post-marketing reports about side effects including depression, suicidal thoughts and suicidal actions. This is, however, controversial and some studies have found no increased risk. It should be used with caution in people with a history of psychiatric illness – depression, bipolar disorder or schizophrenia. Like bupropion it may also increase the risk of seizure and it should be used with caution in people with epilepsy.

It must be borne in mind, however, that every day in the UK there are at least 300 deaths that can be directly attributed to smoking. One in every two life-long smokers will die as a consequence of their habit; very poor odds. Nicotine addiction is difficult to overcome and both bupropion and varenicline are useful weapons in the fight against the addiction. The risks of continuing to smoke far outweigh the risks of using either of these therapies, provided they are given to carefully selected people. World-wide, these medications have helped millions of smokers to stop!

Helping patients to stop smoking

Helping patients to stop smoking can be the most rewarding and the most frustrating of tasks. However, it is the single most important thing you can do to improve the health of your patient. You must ask the smoker about their smoking habits and offer support and advice at every attendance. It is tempting sometimes not to bother to raise the subject because you know that you have discussed smoking cessation with that patient many times and your advice hasn't been heeded. But this may be the one time when you may make a difference. The following hints may be helpful.

Practical hints for health professionals

- Raise the subject of smoking cessation in a non-threatening way.

- Assess motivation to quit by asking open questions such as 'How do you feel about stopping smoking?'

- Show concern and offer appropriate advice/leaflets to the 'contented' smoker.

- Talking about the 'risks' of smoking can be counterproductive. Instead, ask the smoker what they see as the benefits of stopping.

- Make a record of a smoker's reasons for wanting to stop so that you can refer back to it with them.

- Acknowledge that stopping can be difficult, and offer a referral to the NHS Stop Smoking Service. Offer constructive support and advice.

- Make a record of what you have advised, so that you do not repeat yourself and can recap and move forward next time.

- Record what the smoker has said to you. You can use it as a starting point when you next meet!

- Discuss the benefits of nicotine replacement therapy, bupropion and varenicline. Help smokers to select and use their chosen form of treatment correctly.

- If smokers decline to attend an NHS Stop Smoking Service make other arrangements to follow them up during their attempt to quit.

- If they don't succeed, encourage them to work out the reasons why they were unsuccessful this time, discover ways to address those difficulties and try again. However, do not offer a repeat prescription for a pharmacological aid for 6 months, unless there are special circumstances that have led to failure of this attempt.

The key recommendations for health professionals are:

- **Ask** about the smoking status of patients at every opportunity.

- **Advise** all smokers to stop.

- **Assist** those interested in doing so.

- **Arrange** follow-up.

- **Refer** to specialist cessation services.

- **Recommend NRT, buproprion or varenicline** to smokers who want to stop, and provide accurate advice about these treatments.

Practical hints for patients

1 Set a 'quit' date

Stopping smoking is something you need to plan. It is seldom successful if it is undertaken on the spur of the moment.

If you cannot face stopping abruptly it may be possible to use nicotine replacement therapy to help you cut back before stopping – but you do need to be committed to eventually giving up cigarettes completely for this to work and you will need to discuss this strategy with your doctor or nurse.

Before quitting it may be helpful to keep a smoking diary so that danger times can be highlighted and strategies formulated for avoiding them.

Family and friends need to be informed so that they don't put temptation in your way.

2 If at all possible, use the NHS Stop Smoking Service in your area

Success rates are much higher when people have support and the staff of these services are specially trained to give you the best possible chance of stopping. You can find information about the

Stop Smoking Service in your area in the telephone directory and there will be posters and information in places like pharmacies, public libraries and doctor's surgeries. Your doctor or nurse will also have information about the service and will be able to refer you.

If you are unable or don't want to use the NHS Stop Smoking Service take up the offer of support from your doctor or nurse. You might also find it helpful to quit with a friend.

Quit (the smoking quitline) is another helpful resource. The telephone numbers are:

- England: 0800 00 22 00

- Northern Ireland: 02890 663 281

- Scotland: 0800 84 84 84

- Wales: 0800 169 0169 (national number) 0300 1000 069

3 Consider using nicotine replacement therapy, bupropion (Zyban) or varenicline (Champix)

They are not a replacement for your will power but can help you cope with cravings and can double your chances of success. Discuss this with your doctor or nurse.

The pharmaceutical companies that make bupropion, vareniciline and nicotine replacement products include in the packs of treatment 'helpline' information and leaflets to help you quit successfully. Some also provide a special service that you can register with for additional support during your quit attempt.

4 Quit day

On 'quit day' get rid of all cigarettes, lighters and ash trays

5 Cash, not ash

Put aside the money you would have spent on smoking and reward yourself after a week or a fortnight.

6 Avoid replacing cigarettes with extra cups of coffee or tea

Caffeine levels will be increased when you stop smoking and unpleasant side-effects (e.g. headaches) may occur. It is better to drink plenty of water or fruit juice.

7 Cravings are short lived

Try to avoid situations where you would normally smoke. For example, instead of sitting down with a cup of coffee after a meal, get up and do something different. It may be advisable to stay away from the pub or from friends who smoke for the critical first two or three weeks. Alcohol may also weaken your power to resist a cigarette. Work out ways to distract yourself when cravings occur, to occupy you until they pass.

8 Keep a 'nibble box' of raw carrots, celery or some other non-fattening food

Weight gain is common (average weight gain is about 4 kilograms). Don't try to diet and quit smoking at the same time, but do try to avoid sucking sweets and eating fattening foods to overcome your craving for cigarettes. As you begin to feel fitter, try taking up some form of exercise. This will help to keep your weight down and improve your general fitness. Exercising can also distract you from your cravings.

9 Take it one day at a time

Tell yourself 'Today, I am not going to have a cigarette.'

10 If you don't succeed this time – try again!

Work out why you have failed and then try again. Learn from your mistakes.

Further reading

Moore D, Aveyard P, Connock M, Wang D, Fry-Smith A (2009) Effectiveness and safety of nicotine replacement therapy assisted reduction to stop smoking: systematic review and meta-analysis. *British Medical Journal* **338**: b1024

National Institute for Health and Clinical Excellence (2007) *Varenicline for smoking cessation.* NICE Technology Appraisal 123. Available at www.nice.org.uk/TA123

National Institute for Health and Clinical Excellence (2008) *Smoking cessation services in primary care, pharmacies, local authorities, workplaces, particularly for manual working groups, pregnant women and hard to reach communicates.* NICE Public Health Guidance 10. Available at www.nice.org.uk/PH010

Pharmacotherapy

BRONCHODILATORS

Main points

1 Bronchodilators are the most important treatment for symptom relief in COPD.

2 They work by

- decreasing bronchomotor tone
- decreasing lung hyperinflation
- decreasing the work of breathing
- thereby lessening breathlessness and improving exercise capability.

3 They are most appropriately taken by inhalation, and have a rapid onset of action.

4 An inhaler device should be selected that the patient can use effectively. A small number of patients with severe COPD may warrant a nebuliser trial.

5 The patient's inhaler technique should be checked at regular intervals.

6 Short-acting beta-2 agonists (SABA) and antimuscarinics (SAMA) are the usual first line of therapy for breathlessness and are equally efficacious. They can be used up to four times a day. Combining the two types of inhaler may have an additive effect.

7 If symptomatic control is inadequate, adding one of the following should be considered:

- long-acting beta-2 agonists (LABA)
- long-acting anticholinergics (LAMA)
- theophyllines.

8 Two new drugs have recently become available – indacterol, a once daily inhaled LABA, and roflumilast, the first of a new class of oral therapy – the PDE4 inhibitors.

9 Both LABAs and LAMAs have been shown to improve quality of life and reduce the frequency of acute exacerbations. Prescribing a LABA and LAMA together may have an additive effect in some patients.

Bronchodilators are the most important symptomatic treatment in COPD. They decrease breathlessness and improve activity levels. Short-acting inhalers are usually the first line of treatment and can be taken as required or up to four times a day. If symptoms persist and inhaler technique is satisfactory, the addition of one of the long-acting agents should be considered. These have added benefits, such as improving quality of life and reducing the frequency of exacerbations. The latest NICE update suggests that long-acting inhalers should be used at an earlier point and that their addition should depend on the degree of symptoms rather than on the severity of airflow obstruction, based on FEV_1 % predicted.

As discussed in the Assessment chapter (Chapter 6), the efficacy of response to a given bronchodilator should not be based on formal reversibility testing. This may show little change, whereas the patient may have noted a good improvement in their symptoms. Therefore, a bronchodilator should be prescribed for a period of a few weeks and the patient reviewed to assess their symptomatic response. The five questions formulated by Paul Jones are helpful in this respect.

1 Has your treatment made a difference to you?

2 Is your breathing easier in any way?

3 Can you do some things now that you could not do before, or the same but faster?

4 Can you do the same things as before but are now less breathless when you do them?

5 Has your sleep improved?

How do bronchodilators work?

Bronchodilators reverse the increased bronchomotor tone found in the airways of COPD patients by relaxing smooth muscle and thus reducing airway resistance. Their main effect is to reduce the amount of air trapping and hyperinflation that causes the patient to work harder to breathe. Several studies have shown improvements in vital capacity (VC) of 500ml or more, with a similar decrease in residual volume (RV) (see Chapter 5 and Figure 5.11). Hyperinflation is reduced, and it is easier and more comfortable for the patient to breathe. Breathlessness and the effort of breathing are reduced, so patients can walk further.

Beta-2 agonists also promote an increase in mucociliary activity, although the clinical importance of this is unclear. Theophyllines may, in addition, have a small effect on increasing respiratory muscle endurance, but again it is hard to assess whether this is of clinical significance.

Bronchodilator administration

As in asthma, the preferred way to use a bronchodilator is by inhalation. Although oral bronchodilators may be just as effective in providing symptom relief, they have the disadvantages of greater side-effects, potential drug interactions and a slower onset of action.

Metered dose inhalers (MDIs) of short-acting bronchodilators are inexpensive and effective, working rapidly to provide symptom relief. Correct timing and co-ordination can make them difficult to use, and less than 50% of patients can inhale from them effectively. This is especially so in elderly patients, who may have other illnesses such as arthritis or dementia. With repeated tuition, or the addition of a spacer or breath-activated MDI, the proportion of patients able to use MDIs effectively can be greatly increased.

Dry powder devices are simpler to use and equally effective but are more expensive. As in asthma, it is essential that patients are prescribed a device that they can use effectively and are assessed for competence in its use by a trained healthcare professional. Patients should be involved in the initial choice of device.

Short-acting bronchodilators

Short-acting beta-2 agonists (SABA): salbutamol and terbutaline

These drugs have a rapid onset of action (usually within five minutes) and a duration of action of three to four hours. They are recommended for both regular treatment and 'as required' for relief of symptoms. They can also be used before exercise to increase exercise tolerance or to relieve breathlessness. If patients are still symptomatic, the addition of a long-acting bronchodilator should be considered. SABAs are safe to take four times daily.

As with any therapy, success or failure of a given agent should be assessed subjectively, from the point of view of the patient's perceived response over a month of treatment, and perhaps also objectively with lung function if appropriate. Alternatives or additions may then need to be explored.

Short-acting antimuscarinic agent (SAMA): ipratropium

Antimuscarinics work primarily on the cholinergic nerve receptors in the airways and reduce smooth muscle tone thereby causing bronchodilation. They also reduce hyperinflation and the work of breathing. SAMAs have a slower onset of action (15–30 minutes) than SABAs (5 minutes) but the results of most comparative studies suggest that they are equally effective in achieving symptom relief. Indeed, in some they have produced a greater response and a longer duration of bronchodilation. The responses of individual patients to both SAMAs and SABAs should therefore be assessed.

Combined short-acting therapy: salbutamol and ipratropium

The use of a SABA with a SAMA may have an additive effect in some patients. Combined therapy may produce greater improvements in exercise tolerance and a greater degree of bronchodilation than either drug used separately.

Long-acting inhaled bronchodilators

Long-acting beta-2 agonists (LABA): salmeterol, formoterol and indacterol

Salmeterol and formoterol have a duration of action of 12 hours, so they should be taken twice daily and on a regular basis to achieve the optimal effect. The newly launched metered dose inhaler, indacterol, lasts for 24 hours and is taken once daily.

In asthma LABA provide good symptom relief, reduce acute exacerbations and much improve overall quality of life when added to mid to higher doses of inhaled corticosteroids. Their role in COPD has become clarified since the start of this century with good and similar benefits found for both the original LABAs. Comparative trials with indacterol are at an early stage, but a study by Dahl et e.l (2010) against formoterol shows it to be at least as good as other LABAs.

Their effects on lung function are similar to those of SABAs in that there are some increases in FEV_1 and peak flow, larger increases in FVC and falls in residual volume, suggesting reduced hyperinflation. These actions continue for 12 or 24 hours compared with about 4 hours for the short-acting agents. Patients experience reductions in breathlessness but not much change in walking distance. Most importantly there is a significant and sustained improvement in quality of life scores in both the total and symptom domains as judged by the St George's Respiratory Questionnaire. Salmeterol has also been shown to improve breathlessness at night in a study by Mahler. All three LABAs have been shown to reduce exacerbation frequency.

The short-term effects of LABAs are therefore similar to those of short-acting agents in improving lung function. In addition, there seems to be more sustained symptom improvement and significant benefit in health status that does not occur with the short-acting agents. In a review article, Johnson and Rennard offered some possible explanations for the added properties of salmeterol. These observations are based on studies in vitro but may go part way to rationalising the extra properties of LABAs.

Salmeterol seems to protect airway epithelial cells from the damaging effect of bacteria such as *Haemophilus influenzae*. It improves cilial beat frequency and thus improves the clearance of mucus from the lungs. Salmeterol improves neutrophil function in several ways, which may help reduce the frequency of acute exacerbations.

More information is required to relate the clinical importance of these findings but LABAs have a useful role in COPD management, particularly if further studies confirm their ability to extend the time between exacerbations. Like other agents, they should have a clinical trial for four to eight weeks and be continued only if they are beneficial for the individual.

Long-acting antimuscarinic (LAMA): tiotropium

Tiotropium is a long-acting muscarinic blocking agent that comes as either a dry powder or mist inhaler (Respimat), which is taken once daily. It has some shared actions with ipratropium but binds mainly to the M3 airway receptors, which greatly enhances its activity and duration of action to 24 hours compared with 4–6 hours for ipratropium.

A one-year study against placebo (Casaburi et al. 2002) confirmed worthwhile improvements in FEV_1, FVC and peak flow throughout the study period. Breathlessness was reduced and health status improved, 49% of patients on active therapy achieving at least a 4-point clinically meaningful increase on the overall score with the St George's Respiratory Questionnaire. There was a 14% reduction in exacerbations compared with placebo and a 47% reduction in hospitalisations. The time to first exacerbation was also significantly longer. A similar one year study against ipratropium obtained comparable results.

A study adding tiotropium before and during pulmonary rehabilitation significantly enhanced the exercise ability and quality of life scores compared with a placebo arm.

The UPLIFT study

The major tiotropium study, UPLIFT (Tashkin et al. 2008), followed a total of 5,993 patients with moderate or severe COPD for 4 years. Patients were allowed all other respiratory medications except ipratropium. The main outcomes were an improvement in FEV_1 of 87–103 ml compared with placebo. The rate of decline in lung function was not different for the full study but a sub analysis in patients with moderate COPD did show a significant decrease in the tiotropium arm – 43ml/year versus 49ml/year in placebo. There were also significant improvements in quality of life scores and a reduction in the number of exacerbations (14%), hospitalisations and respiratory failure.

If a trial of LAMA is successful, any SAMA the patient is taking should be stopped.

Combined LABAs and LAMAs

The NICE Guideline update has suggested that the two groups of long-acting bronchodilators can be used together for more severe symptomatic breathlessness, although it is more likely that, at this stage an inhaled corticosteroid would also be added to make a triple therapy. The evidence base for LABA plus LAMA versus LAMA alone demonstrates little added benefit in terms of lung function and exacerbations, but the quality of life improvement was greater for the combined therapy.

Oral long-acting bronchodilators

Beta-2 agonists

Generally these agents are not encouraged, as the inhaled versions work more rapidly and are safer. However, they may occasionally be justified for a patient with severe COPD who has difficulty using any form of inhaled therapy. If they are used, care must be taken to ensure that there is no significant side-effect such as tremor, tachycardia or hypokalaemia and that coexisting angina is not being made worse.

Theophyllines

Theophyllines produce only small amounts of bronchodilation in COPD and tend to be most effective in the higher parts of the narrow therapeutic range (i.e. blood levels of 10–20mg/litre). They can increase exercise tolerance, and some patients report a good improvement in symptoms. Other effects reported in research studies – such as an anti-inflammatory action, improvements in respiratory muscle strength and improvements in right ventricular performance – are difficult to evaluate clinically. If theophyllines are used, it is preferable to give them in a slow-release form, and to monitor serum theophylline levels regularly.

Side-effects such as nausea, headache and palpitations are common and there are also interactions with anti-epileptic drugs, diltiazem, verapamil, frusemide, erythromycin, ciprofloxacin and cimetidine, to name but a few. Blood levels are also influenced by smoking, viral infections, influenza vaccination and impaired renal and hepatic function. In elderly patients with multiple co-pathologies it can be extremely difficult to achieve an effective and stable blood level of theophylline. The risk/benefit ratio must therefore be considered carefully.

Theophyllines can be added to inhaled bronchodilators in more severe COPD.

Phosphodiesterase inhibitors (PDE4 inhibitors): Roflumilast

Phosphodiesterases are a family of enzymes found in all parts of the body. In the lung they have an important role in the airways. They work to increase the amount of cyclic AMP (cyclic adenosine monophosphate), which has a major role in airway smooth muscle relaxation, and also suppresses many parts of the inflammatory cascade, particularly neutrophils.

Theophyllines fall into this group of drugs but act on many phosphodiesterases in other parts of the body, like the heart and brain, resulting in possible significant side effects. The new class of PDE4 inhibitors is much more specific to actions in the lung and thus has fewer side effects.

Roflumilast is a once daily oral drug that was launched in late 2010. The clinical patient group for its use are more severe patients with chronic bronchitis who are having exacerbations. Clinical trials have shown a small increase in FEV_1 of 48ml compared with placebo, some improvement in breathlessness and a 17% reduction in exacerbations. Studies on quality of life did not reach significance.

Roflumilast can be added to other therapy such as LABAs and LAMAs with additive effect. More studies are needed to fully establish the role and efficacy of this new drug.

Nebulised bronchodilators

A small number of patients with severe COPD do not show any symptomatic improvement with inhaled bronchodilators, even with multiple doses taken through a spacer. Sometimes benefit can be achieved only by using higher doses via a nebuliser. Nebulised bronchodilators are generally more expensive. They are also less convenient to administer because they take longer and a power source is usually required, although some nebuliser/compressor systems have rechargeable battery packs or run off a car cigarette lighter thus allowing the patient greater flexibility and mobility.

Nebuliser therapy

Nebulisers are devices that convert a drug solution into a fine aerosol of sufficiently small particle size to penetrate to all levels of the airways. Drug inhalation is achieved by the patient breathing normally (tidal breathing) through the nebuliser over a five to ten minute period. The advantage of a nebuliser is that it can deliver a large dose of drug simply, particularly to patients who are too breathless or unwell to use a normal inhaler device effectively, or who have benefited clinically from higher doses.

The most commonly used varieties of nebuliser are:

- the standard jet nebuliser

- the more advanced and efficient breath-assisted nebulisers, such as the Ventstream

- the ultrasonic nebuliser

- the mesh nebuliser.

The first two of these need to be driven by a compressor delivering flow rates of 6–8 litres per minute. Adaptive aerosol delivery, delivers the drug during inhalation only, thus eliminating waste of drug during exhalation, and can be programmed to deliver a precise dose. It costs more than both the standard nebuliser/compressor system and the ultrasonic nebuliser. If delivery of a precise amount of drug is not of paramount importance, it may not be a cost-effective option.

Ultrasonic and mesh nebuliser systems are smaller and operate almost silently. They are only suitable for single-patient use and are a little more expensive than the jet nebuliser systems. However, for a patient who requires a small, discreet system that is easy to use outside the home, these may be an attractive option.

The ultrasonic nebuliser uses ultrasound to agitate the drug solution so that droplets of appropriate size break off the surface. In the mesh system, drug solution is forced through microscopic holes in a metal mesh, forming respirable droplets of the solution. The mesh system is completely silent and very quick and efficient.

A mouthpiece is usually preferred to a facemask to deliver the nebulised mist. This is because there is a small risk of precipitating glaucoma when ipratropium or a combination of ipratropium and salbutamol is used via a facemask.

If a nebuliser/compressor system is supplied for long-term use at home, patients and their carers need to be given written instructions about cleaning and maintaining the equipment. Nebuliser chamber and mouthpiece or facemask need to be washed in warm soapy water and dried thoroughly after each use. The small jet holes in a jet nebuliser can be dried by attaching the nebuliser to the compressor and running the compressor for about ten seconds to remove any residual fluid. Standard disposable nebuliser chambers will last a single patient for three months of regular use before they become inefficient and need to be replaced. Tubing should not be washed inside because it is impossible to dry it effectively. Nebuliser equipment that is stored damp may constitute an infection risk.

Compressors need to be serviced regularly, according to manufacturer's instructions. An annual electrical safety check is the legal responsibility of whoever supplies the compressor.

In the surgery, standard nebulisers, tubing and masks are for single use only and should then be discarded. It is not possible to sterilise them effectively and there is thus a risk of passing infection from one patient to another. For medico-legal purposes, it is advisable to adhere to the single-use policy. 'Durable' nebulisers are made by some manufacturers; these can be sterilised effectively in an autoclave and used for a year. They may be more cost-effective than single-use disposable nebulisers. Maintenance of equipment should follow the manufacturer's recommendations.

Nebuliser trials

The BTS *Nebuliser Guidelines* require patients to attempt high-dose bronchodilator therapy through a spacer before undertaking a formal nebuliser trial. Up to six to eight 'puffs' of bronchodilator are given through a spacer, with the patient inhaling each puff separately, 4-hourly. Assessment for the appropriate use of a nebuliser should follow BTS

Guidelines for nebuliser therapy and be carried out by a hospital specialist or a GP with experience of nebuliser trials. Nebulised beta-2 agonists and antimuscarinics should be tried alone and then in combination in order to determine which therapy produces the best effect.

To perform a nebuliser trial the patient should be clinically stable. A suggested protocol is:

- Weeks 1–2: spacer and high-dose bronchodilator

- Weeks 3–4: nebulised short-acting beta-2 agonist (e.g. salbutamol 2.5–5mg or terbutaline 5–10mg four times a day)

- Weeks 5–6: nebulised antimuscarinic (e.g. ipratropium bromide 250–500 mg four times a day)

- Weeks 7–8: nebulised combined short-acting beta-2 agonist and antimuscarinic (e.g. salbutamol 5mg + ipratropium 500 mg four times a day).

Patients should perform serial peak flow tests during the trial. A positive response is either an increase in lung function (improvement of 15% in peak flow during the trial) or a definite improvement in symptoms on active treatment. If a nebuliser is helpful, a nebuliser/compressor unit should be provided by the local chest clinic, who will:

- educate the patient and their carer(s) in its use

- provide regular maintenance of the unit

- supply disposables such as the nebuliser chamber

- provide emergency back-up in the event of breakdown.

Unfortunately, the provision of properly organised, hospital-based nebuliser services remains patchy. In many areas of the UK, patients (or their GPs) are expected to purchase and maintain nebulisers for long-term use. This situation is far from satisfactory.

Bronchodilator therapy can improve a COPD patient's symptoms without necessarily producing significant changes in lung function. All patients should undergo therapeutic trials with different bronchodilators and different combinations of bronchodilators at different doses in order to determine which drug (or drugs) produces the best therapeutic response.

Further reading

General

British Thoracic Society (1997) Current best practice for nebuliser treatment. *Thorax* **52** (Suppl 2): S1–106

National Clinical Guideline Centre (2010) Chronic obstructive pulmonary disease: the management of chronic obstructive pulmonary disease in adults in primary and secondary care. London. CG101. Available at http://guidance.nice.org.uk/CG101/Guidance/pdf/English

Nisar M, Walshaw M, Earis JE, Pearson M, Calverley PMA (1990) Assessment of reversibility of airway obstruction in patients with chronic obstructive airways disease. *Thorax* **45**: 190–4

Calverley PMA, Burge PS, Spencer S, et al. (2003) Bronchodilator reversibility testing in chronic obstructive pulmonary disease. *Thorax* **58**: 659–64

Short-acting beta-2 agonists

Bellamy D, Hutchison DCS (1981) The effects of salbutamol aerosol on the lung function of patients with emphysema. *British Journal of Diseases of the Chest* **75**: 190–5

van Schayck CP, Dompeling E, van Herwaarden CLA, Folgering H, Verbeek AL, van der Hoogen HJ (1991) Bronchodilator treatment in moderate asthma or chronic bronchitis; continuous or on demand. A randomised controlled study. *British Medical Journal* **303**: 1426–31

Short-acting antimuscarinics

Anthonisen NR, Connett JE, Kiley JP, et al. (1994) Effects of smoking intervention and the use of an inhaled anticholinergic bronchodilator on the rate of decline of FEV_1. *Journal of the American Medical Association* **272**: 1497–505

Braun SR, McKenzie WN, Copeland C, Knight I, Ellersieck M (1989) A comparison of the effect of ipratropium and albuterol in the treatment of chronic airways disease. *Archives of Internal Medicine* **149**: 544–7

Combivent Inhalation Aerosol Study (1994) Combination of ipratropium and albuterol is more effective than either agent alone. *Chest* **105**: 1411–19

Long-acting beta-2 agonists

Appleton S, Poole P, Smith B, et al. (2006) Long-acting beta-2 agonists for poorly reversible chronic obstructive pulmonary disease. *Cochrane Database of Systemic Reviews* 2006 Issue 3.

Boyd G, Morice AH, Poundsford JC, Siebert M, Peslis N, Crawford C (1997) An evaluation of salmeterol in the treatment of chronic obstructive airways disease. *European Respiratory Journal* 10: 815–21

Dahl R, Chung KF, Buhl, et al. (2010) Efficacy of a new once daily long-acting inhaled beta-2 agonist indacterol versus twice-daily formoterol in COPD. *Thorax* 65: 473–9

Johnson M, Rennard S (2001) Alternative mechanisms for long-acting beta-2-adrenergic agonists in COPD. *Chest* 120: 258–70

Jones PW, Bosh TK (1997) Quality of life changes in COPD patients treated with salmeterol. *American Journal of Respiratory and Critical Care Medicine* 155: 1283–9

Mahler DA, Donohue JF, Barbee RA, et al. (1999) Efficacy of salmeterol in the treatment of COPD. *Chest* 115: 957–65

Long-acting antimuscarinincs

Casaburi R, Mahler DA, Jones PW, et al. (2002) A long-term evaluation of once-daily inhaled tiotropium in chronic obstructive pulmonary disease. *European Respiratory Journal* 19: 217–24

Decramer M, Celli B, Kesten S, et al. (2009) Effect of tiotropium on outcomes in patients with moderate chronic obstructive pulmonary disease (UPLIFT): a pre-specified subgroup analysis of a randomised controlled trial. *Lancet* 374: 1171–8.

Littner MR, Ilowite JS, Tashkin DA, et al. (2000) Long-acting bronchodilation with once daily dosing of tiotropium in stable COPD. *American Journal of Respiratory and Critical Care Medicine* 161: 1136–42

Tashkin DP, Celli B, Senn S, et al. (2008) A 4 year trial of tiotropium in chronic obstructive pulmonary disease. (UPLIFT study.) *New England Journal of Medicine* 359: 1543–54

Van Noord JA, Bantje TA, Eland ME, et al. (2000) A randomised controlled comparison of tiotropium and ipratropium in the treatment of COPD. *Thorax* 55: 289–94

Vincken W, van Noord APM, Greefhorst TA, et al. (2002) Improved health outcomes in patients with COPD during 1year's treatment with tiotropium. *European Respiratory Journal* **19**: 209–16

Theophyllines

McKay SE, Howie CA, Thomson AH, Whiting B, Addis GJ (1993) Value of theophylline treatment in patients handicapped by chronic obstructive pulmonary disease. *Thorax* **48**: 227–32

PDE4 inhibitors

Calverley PMA, Rabe KF, Goehring U, et al. (2009) Roflumilast in symptomatic chronic obstructive pulmonary disease: two trials. *Lancet* **374**: 685–94
Fabbri LM, Calverley PMA, Izquierdo-Alonso JL, et al. (2009) Roflumilast in moderate-to-severe chronic obstructive pulmonary disease treated with long-acting bronchodilators: two randomised clinical trials. *Lancet* **374**; 695–703

CORTICOSTEROID THERAPY

Main points

1 Inflammatory changes exist in the airways and connective tissues of patients with COPD, with increases of neutrophils, T-lymphocytes and macrophages. There is also tissue and alveolar destruction and increased mucous production. These inflammatory changes are different from those in asthma.

2 The effect of inhaled corticosteroids on the cells and mediators in the airways has been studied with bronchoscopic biopsies and induced sputum. Generally there are little or no responses with up to 3 months of high-dose inhaled corticosteroid.

3 Corticosteroid reversibility testing is infrequently needed but if there is diagnostic doubt a trial of prednisolone 30mg per day for two weeks should be done – an increase greater than 400ml in FEV_1 is suggestive of asthma.

4 GOLD guidelines prefer corticosteroid reversibility testing with 6–12 weeks of inhaled beclomethasone 1000 µg/day (or equivalent). Reversibility is assessed by a 12% increase and 200ml improvement in FEV_1.

5 Clinical trials of various inhaled corticosteroids have shown an initial improvement in lung function which may be maintained, but no effect on decline in FEV_1. More recent trials such as TORCH, however, have suggested a small benefit in FEV_1 decline.

6 All major guidelines suggest that patients with moderate or severe COPD – FEV_1 less than 50% predicted – and who are having regular exacerbations should be treated with long-term high-dose inhaled corticosteroids. In the NICE 2010 update this has been extended to patients with milder disease who have inadequately controlled symptoms and regular exacerbations.

7 There is little evidence to use inhaled corticosteroids in patients with mild disease unless they are having frequent exacerbations.

8 The main benefits of inhaled corticosteroids are improvement of symptoms, reduction in the frequency of exacerbations (about 25%) and slowing of health status deterioration with time.

9 Recent studies have shown a small increased risk of pneumonia with any treatments containing inhaled corticosteroids. There is likely to be increased risk of cataracts but the effect on higher prevalence of osteoporosis may be largely due to the COPD itself.

10 Inhaled corticosteroids are not licensed for use on their own in COPD. Combined inhalers with LABAs, however, are a very effective treatment.

11 The new NICE flow chart for bronchodilator and inhaled corticosteroid treatment is shown in Figure 8.1.

In asthma, there is abundant evidence that the chronic inflammatory changes in the mucosa of the airways can be made histologically normal with both oral and inhaled corticosteroids. However, although the symptoms of most patients with COPD will improve with bronchodilator therapy, their response to corticosteroids is far less clear-cut. The chronic inflammatory changes in the airways have been studied with bronchoscopic biopsies and from induced sputum after 3 months of high-dose inhaled corticosteroids. Disappointingly there have been very small or no changes in the cells or inflammatory mediators. We know that COPD is a spectrum of diseases with chronic bronchitis, emphysema and long-standing asthma that has become poorly reversible. Little has been done to assess treatment in these clinical phenotypes. It might be anticipated that the bronchitic/asthmatic type of patient with greater levels of reversibility might respond better to corticosteroids.

The NICE guidelines advice on inhaled corticosteroids in COPD

Oral corticosteroid reversibility tests do not predict response to inhaled corticosteroid therapy and should not be used to identify which patients should be prescribed inhaled corticosteroids. When there is diagnostic doubt, a trial of prednisolone 30mg per day for two weeks should be done – an increase greater than 400ml in FEV_1 is suggestive of asthma.

Previously it was recommended that inhaled corticosteroids be prescribed for patients with an FEV_1 less than or equal to 50% predicted who had had two or more exacerbations in the last year. The aim of treatment was to reduce exacerbations and slow the rate of decline in health status, and not to slow the rate of decline in lung function. The 2010 update has extended inhaled corticosteroid use to patients with a FEV_1 greater than 50% who are symptomatic and having regular exacerbations. Figure 8.1 based on the NICE update summarises the flow of symptomatic treatment for bronchodilators and corticosteroids.

Several major clinical trials such as the TORCH study have found an increased level of pneumonia in patients who are taking therapies with inhaled corticosteroids. There is also a potential risk of osteoporosis but this does not appear to be of much clinical significance over and above the much higher prevalence linked with COPD itself.

Use of inhaled therapies

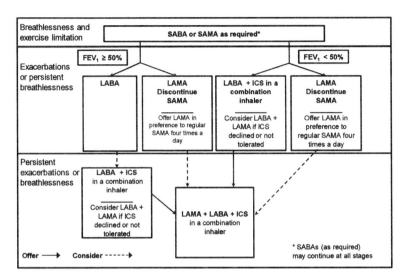

Figure 8.1 NICE update 2010 – treatment pathways for bronchodilators and steroids

The main actions of inhaled corticosteroids in COPD

Since the mid-1990s, a number of major studies have clarified the clinical role of inhaled corticosteroids. There is strong evidence that they:

- reduce the frequency of exacerbations – by about 20–25%

- improve symptoms and quality of life

- improve lung function initially and maintain some improvement longer term

- slow the decline in quality of life with time

- have little benefit in patients with mild disease.

These effects have been established with high doses of inhaled corticosteroids only.

There is more debate around actions related to changes in the decline in FEV_1 and all cause mortality. A post-hoc analysis from the

TORCH study (2008) calculated a small but significant reduction in decline in FEV$_1$ in all the active treatment arms, which included fluticasone on its own. Two studies by Sin (2001, 2005) analysed deaths in previous major studies and found that all cause mortality was decreased by 27% (2005 study) in the active treatment arm compared to placebo. The statistical methodology of these studies has been questioned by experts and none of the studies analysed had deaths as one of their outcome measures.

Summary of important messages from major inhaled corticosteroid studies

- In the short term, there are clinically significant improvements in lung function and symptoms, with fewer acute exacerbations. The results from the Isolde study indicate that improvements are maintained for three years.

- There is relatively little or no change in the rate of decline of lung function (FEV$_1$) over three years with various inhaled corticosteroids in moderate to high dosage (Euroscop, Isolde, Copenhagen Lung Study, Lung Health 2 and the 1999 meta-analysis).

- Two meta-analyses (Highland et al. 2003, Sutherland et al. 2003), essentially analysing the same data from six studies, concluded that inhaled corticosteroids, particularly in higher dose over two years had a small beneficial effect by reducing the rate of decline in FEV$_1$ by 9.9ml per year compared with placebo. The study by Highland et al., found the benefit to be only 5ml per year, which was not statistically significant. Where does this guide us? The inference is that inhaled corticosteroids in high dosage may have a small benefit on reducing the rate of decline in lung function but seemingly not in milder cases.

- The decline in quality of life is significantly slowed over a 3-year period by high-dose fluticasone (Isolde).

- The dose of inhaled corticosteroid in everyday practice is uncertain but needs to be in the higher range – beclomethasone 1000–2000 µg/day, fluticasone 500–1000 µg/day.

What are the implications for primary care?

The benefits on reducing decline in lung function are small. There may be an effect on reducing mortality particularly in combination with LABAs and/or LAMAs and this could be mediated through the effect on reducing exacerbation frequency. However, there is strong evidence for the improvements in exacerbation frequency, symptoms and quality of life. These effects are of considerable importance to patients.

Oral corticosteroids: what is their role?

Most GP practices have patients with severe COPD who take oral corticosteroids, usually for acute exacerbations. However, because of the potential side-effects, the NICE guidelines do not recommend the regular use of oral corticosteroids. When these are gradually stopped, the patient may deteriorate rapidly, with worsening dyspnoea, cough or wheeze. So a further course of corticosteroids is given. If the symptoms become worse as the steroids are again reduced, this usually indicates the need for ongoing oral corticosteroid therapy. Such circumstances usually guide the decision to continue oral corticosteroids unless or until their side-effects outweigh the benefits. Each patient needs to be counselled about the advantages and disadvantages of this therapy in relation to the severity of their disease, likely benefits and the side-effects, and should be involved in the decision whether to continue.

The likelihood of serious side-effects is fairly small when a low dose of oral corticosteroids is used. Each patient should be observed carefully for reduced mobility due to muscle weakness in the thighs from corticosteroid myopathy.

A number of guidelines have appeared relating to the increased risk of bone fracture with oral corticosteroids. Vertebral fractures are more likely to occur than limb fractures; they are related to the corticosteroid dose but also to risk factors particular to the individual patient. As the greatest rate of bone loss seems to happen in the first 12 months of treatment, early steps to prevent osteoporosis are important.

One of the guidelines uses a dose of 5mg of prednisolone per day as a cut-off point and recommends that bone mineral density be measured by dexa-scan above this threshold. Recommended treatment is with bisphosphonates, which significantly increase bone density but, according to a Cochrane review, do not reduce overall fractures.

Corticosteroids for acute exacerbations

It is common practice in primary and secondary care to treat exacerbations of COPD with courses of prednisolone, particularly when the symptoms are increasing breathlessness, wheeze and chest tightness. Symptoms usually return to baseline levels over one to three weeks and, as with acute asthma, the corticosteroid treatment may need to be continued for up to 14 days.

Do corticosteroids have particular side-effects in COPD?

The side-effects of inhaled and systemic corticosteroids are summarised in Table 8.1. Four factors are of particular relevance in COPD:

1 Patients are generally older.
2 They have severe COPD with multiple exacerbations and usually limited life expectancy.
3 There may be co-morbidities and other chronic diseases.
4 Most receive a relatively small maintenance dose of oral corticosteroids.

Table 8.1 Side-effects of corticosteroids

Inhaled	*Systemic*
Oral candidiasis	Suppressed hypothalamic–pituitary–adrenal function
Dysphonia	Osteoporosis
Bruising	Hypertension
Cataracts	Cataracts
Pneumonia	Weight gain
?Osteoporosis	Dyspepsia
	Cushingoid appearance
	Mood change
	Peripheral oedema
	Risk of diabetes
	Myopathy

Inhaled corticosteroids seem to cause only minor side-effects, apart from mild oral and laryngeal problems and an increased risk of bruising. Oral corticosteroids cause suppression of pituitary–adrenal function but this side-effect is probably of little clinical importance. Perhaps the main concern in severe COPD is the potential added effect on bone thinning from smoking and inactivity. Unfortunately, there have not been any controlled studies that specifically addressed these questions.

Synopsis of important clinical trials of inhaled corticosteroids in COPD

Short-term trials

The study of Dompeling et al. (1992) examined a mixed group of asthma and COPD patients with known more rapid decline in lung function than usual. All patients were treated for a year with beclometasone 800 μg daily together with either salbutamol or ipratropium. In the patients with COPD there was a significant improvement in the rate of decline of FEV_1 in the first six months of treatment, but from months 7–12 the rate of decline returned to pre-steroid treatment levels. There was no change in the number of exacerbations but a small improvement in the symptoms of cough, sputum and dyspnoea. This study thus suggests small improvements in symptoms and slowed rate of decline in FEV_1 in the first six months that subsequently revert to pre-corticosteroid treatment levels.

The two-year study by Renkema et al. (1996) examined 58 non-allergic patients with COPD. They were given:

- budesonide 1600 μg per day, or
- budesonide 1600 μg per day plus oral prednisolone 5mg per day, or
- a placebo.

As with the Dompeling study, there was a small but significant improvement in symptoms but no change in the number of exacerbations. The rate of decline of FEV_1 was:

- budesonide only: 30ml per year,

- budesonide plus prednisolone: 40ml per year,

- placebo: 60ml per year.

Because of a wide scatter of results, none of the differences reached statistical significance. The authors concluded that, over all, the benefits of the corticosteroids were small but that some patients might achieve worthwhile responses. More studies are required to determine which COPD patients should receive inhaled corticosteroids.

A multi-centre study by Paggiaro et al. (1998) compared fluticasone 1000 µg per day with a placebo in 281 patients over a six-month period. These patients generally had more severe COPD than those in the studies described above. Outcome measures were symptom scores, exacerbations and lung function. Compared with the placebo group, the active treatment group had:

- fewer exacerbations ($p < 0.001$)

- improved symptom scores

- a greater walking distance

- improved peak flow and FEV_1.

This study also indicates a short-term improvement with inhaled corticosteroids, but the dose of fluticasone was high and probably more than would customarily be used in general practice. We do not know whether this response would have continued if the study had been extended although a longer study, Isolde, gives some indication (see later).

In complete contrast, a study from Canada by Bourbeau et al. (1998) has shown no response to budesonide 1600 µg per day over six months. This was also a placebo-controlled trial but the patients included had severe, advanced COPD. Initially, all patients received prednisolone 40mg per day for two weeks, and only those who were deemed corticosteroid non-responders entered the double-blind phase of the study. Only 13.5% of the original 140 patients were designated corticosteroid responders. There were no differences in FEV_1, symptom scores or quality of life scores between the treatment and the placebo groups.

These studies help to demonstrate the difficulty in interpreting the efficacy of inhaled corticosteroids and the importance of knowing the selection criteria for the patients studied. The Dompeling study had patients with milder COPD; moreover, some of them were atopic and thus more likely to respond to the corticosteroid. Over all, though, there seems to be a favourable short-term effect on symptoms in the first six months. The longer term changes in the rate of decline of lung function are, however, minimal.

Longer term studies

Two early studies by Postma (1985, 1988) reviewed retrospectively a group of patients with severe COPD for between 2 and 20 years. The patients who had regularly been taking oral prednisolone 10mg or more per day had a slower decline in FEV_1. If, however, the dose of prednisolone was reduced to less than 10mg per day, the FEV_1 tended to fall more rapidly. It is therefore important to balance the clinical benefits with the likely increasing number of side-effects from oral corticosteroid therapy. At present, only patients with severe COPD would be considered for long-term oral corticosteroids.

Multi-centre studies

Three major multi-centre studies were completed in the 1990s. Each addressed the longer term effect of inhaled corticosteroids on the decline of lung function compared with a control group.

Euroscop (Pauwels et al. 1999) was a large European placebo-controlled study examining the effect of budesonide 800 µg per day on the rate of decline of lung function over a three-year period. Entry criteria to the study included being a current smoker with a FEV_1/FVC ratio less than 70% and less than 10% reversibility following a course of prednisolone. Initially, 2147 people were recruited; those who stopped smoking or were non-compliant during the run-in period were dropped from the study, leaving 1277 participants. They had a mean age of 52 years and a mean FEV_1% predicted of 77% – mild COPD. The primary outcome variable was post-bronchodilator FEV_1.

The results revealed relatively small differences between the two groups. The overall three-year decline in FEV_1 was 140ml in the budesonide group and 180ml in the placebo group.

As in other studies, there was an initial improvement over the first six months with the inhaled corticosteroid, followed by a similar decline from 9 to 36 months. Subgroup analysis revealed that:

- women did better than men

- heavier smokers declined more rapidly

- atopy had no significant role.

The overall conclusion was that the inhaled corticosteroid had a limited long-term benefit on the rate of decline in lung function.

Isolde (Burge et al. 2000) This British study compared fluticasone 500 μg twice daily (via MDI and large volume spacer) with a placebo in moderate to severe COPD over a three-year period. The participants were older (mean age 64) and heavy smokers (44 pack-years). Outcome measures were:

- post-bronchodilator FEV_1

- frequency of exacerbations

- withdrawal from the study for respiratory reasons

- health status scores.

After a two-month run-in period to obtain baseline levels, participants were given an oral prednisolone challenge and then randomised to fluticasone (376 patients, of whom 216 completed) or placebo (375 patients, of whom 180 completed). The mean FEV_1% predicted was 50% with corticosteroid reversibility of 6%.

The difference in the *total rate of decline of FEV$_1$* over the three years was greater than in the Euroscop study, with values of 133ml for the fluticasone group and 197ml for the placebo group (p = 0.0003). In the fluticasone group, the improvement peaked at six to nine months. Thereafter the annual decline in FEV_1 was fairly similar at 50ml for fluticasone and 59ml for placebo.

Exacerbation rates were lower on fluticasone (0.99 per year vs 1.32 on placebo) and there were more *withdrawals for respiratory causes* in the placebo group.

Health status was assessed using the St George's Questionnaire, which correlates well with respiratory symptoms but less well with FEV_1. A significant clinical change on this scale corresponds to four 'units'. Participants receiving fluticasone had a significantly slower rate of decline in health status than did those on placebo. A deterioration of four units occurred every 15 months in the placebo group, against 24 months in the fluticasone group. Thus, in this study of patients with moderate to severe COPD, high-dose fluticasone resulted in fewer exacerbations, improved symptoms and a better quality of life throughout the period of the study. The effect on the rate of decline in lung function was small, particularly over the last two years of the study. The run-in phase of this study showed that a conventional oral corticosteroid trial was a poor predictor of the response to long-term inhaled corticosteroid therapy.

Copenhagen Lung Study (Vestbo et al. 1999) This three-year Danish study compared budesonide 800 µg per day (via turbohaler) with a placebo. The patients recruited for it had very mild impairment of lung function (FEV_1% predicted 86%); indeed, many of them would not match the original BTS (1997) Guidelines definition of COPD or the current NICE (2010) criteria. However, they were all heavy smokers. Out of 416 patients, 395 had no response to an initial trial with prednisolone.

At the end of the study, the decline in FEV_1 was almost identical: 46ml per year for the group receiving budesonide and 49ml per year for the placebo group – indicating no significant clinical benefit from budesonide over three years. However, the selection of corticosteroid non-responders and an initial six months of high-dose budesonide would minimise any effect.

Lung Health 2 Study (2000) This large study from the USA enrolled 1116 patients with milder COPD (mean FEV_1 of 68% predicted) and treated them with the inhaled corticosteroid triamcinolone or a placebo for three years. The dose used was lower than that used in other studies. As with the other studies, there was no effect on the rate of decline of FEV_1 between the treatment groups. However, patients in the triamcinolone group had fewer respiratory symptoms and fewer visits to a respiratory physician. The side-effects were carefully monitored and revealed that the bone density in the corticosteroid group decreased during the study. Triamcinolone is, however, recognised as a less selective inhaled corticosteroid and is not used in this format in the UK.

Inhaled corticosteroid meta-analysis (Van Grunsven et al. 1999) This combined Dutch–French meta-analysis looked at the effects of inhaled corticosteroids in placebo-controlled trials over a two-year period. It identified three studies – two published and one in abstract form – and reanalysed the original data to conform to a more uniform format. Patients were included only if they had definite COPD.

The results show a small improvement in FEV_1 of 34ml per year in favour of the group receiving inhaled corticosteroids. There was no difference in exacerbation rates in the two groups. The patients in the studies using high-dose corticosteroids (beclometasone 1500 μg per day) did better than those on lower doses (budesonide 800 μg per day), in whom there was little effect.

The authors of the paper conclude that this is the first published study to show a preservation of FEV_1 during two years of treatment, but only with high doses of inhaled corticosteroid. This important study adds weight to the provisional early reports from the Isolde study that high-dose inhaled corticosteroids seem to have a beneficial effect on long-term COPD; lower doses apparently do not.

Sin (2005) pooled data from the four major studies and three others and examined 5,085 patients followed for over a year with the major outcome being all cause mortality. In none of these studies was death an end point. He found a 27% reduction in all cause mortality in the corticosteroid treated patients, with women, ex-smokers and more severe patients doing best. There are some limitations to this study and other experts have criticised the statistical methods used.

Despite 15 years of study there is still much argument about some of the roles of inhaled corticosteroids in COPD. These have been aired in a recent editorial pro/con debate (Postma and Calverley 2009, Suissa and Barnes, 2009).

Further reading

General

National Clinical Guideline Centre (2010) *Chronic obstructive pulmonary disease: the management of chronic obstructive pulmonary disease in adults in primary and secondary care.* London. CG101. Available at http://guidance.nice.org.uk/CG101/Guidance/pdf/English

Common issues in osteoporosis. *MeReC Bulletin* (2001) **12**: 5–8

Jarad NA, Wedzicha JA, Burge PS, et al. (1999) An observational study of inhaled corticosteroid withdrawal in stable chronic obstructive pulmonary disease. *Respiratory Medicine* **93**: 161–6

McEvoy CE, Niewoehner DE (1997) Adverse effects of corticosteroid therapy for COPD – a critical review. *Chest* **111**: 732–43

Postma DS, Calverley P (2009) Inhaled corticosteroids in COPD: a case in favour. *European Respiratory Journal* **34**: 10–12

Royal College of Physicians of Edinburgh (2001) *Consensus Statement on the Management of COPD.* RCPE, Edinburgh [Available on-line (contact details in the 'Useful addresses' section)]

Sin DD, Tu JV (2001) Inhaled corticosteroids and the risk of mortality and readmission in elderly patients with COPD. *American Journal of Respiratory and Critical Care Medicine* **164**: 580–4

Suissa S, Barnes PJ (2009) Inhaled corticosteroids in COPD; the case against. *European Respiratory Journal* **34**: 13–16

Thompson WH, Nielson CP, Carvalho P et al. (1996) Controlled trial of oral prednisolone in outpatients with acute COPD exacerbation. *American Journal of Respiratory and Critical Care Medicine* **154**: 407–12

Short-term trials

Bourbeau J, Rouleau MY, Boucher S (1998) Randomised controlled trial of inhaled corticosteroids in patients with COPD. *Thorax* **53**: 447–82

Dompeling E, van Schayk CP, Molema J, et al. (1992) Inhaled beclometasone improves the course of asthma and COPD. *European Respiratory Journal* **5**: 945–52

Paggiaro PL, Dahle R, Bakran I, et al. (1998) Multicentre randomised placebo controlled trial of inhaled fluticasone in patients with COPD. *Lancet* **351**: 773–9

Renkema TEJ, Schouten MS, Koeter GH, Postma DS (1996) Effects of long term treatment with corticosteroids in COPD. *Chest* **109**: 1156–62

Long-term trials

Burge PS, Calverley PMA, Jones PW, et al. (2000) Randomised, double-blind, placebo-controlled study of fluticasone propionate in patients with moderate to severe chronic obstructive pulmonary disease: the Isolde trial. *British Medical Journal* **320**: 1297–303

Lung Health Study Research Group (2000) Effect of inhaled triamcinolone on the decline in pulmonary function in COPD. *New England Journal of Medicine* **343**: 1902–9

Pauwels RA, Lofdahl C, Laitinen LA, et al. (1999) Long-term treatment with inhaled budesonide in persons with mild chronic obstructive pulmonary disease who continue smoking. *New England Journal of Medicine* **340**: 1948–53

Postma DS, Steenhuis EJ, Vanderweele LT, et al. (1985) Severe chronic airflow obstruction: can corticosteroids slow down progression? *European Journal of Respiratory Disease* **67**: 56–64

Postma DS, Peters I, Steenhuis EJ, et al. (1988) Moderately severe chronic airflow obstruction: can corticosteroids slow down progression? *European Respiratory Journal* **1**: 22–6

Vestbo J, Sorensen T, Lange P, et al. (1999) Long-term effects of inhaled budesonide in mild and moderate chronic obstructive pulmonary disease: a randomised controlled trial. *Lancet* **353**: 1819–23

Meta-analysis

Highland KB, Strange C, Heffner JE (2003) Long-term effects of inhaled corticosteroids on FEV_1 in patients with COPD. A meta-analysis. *Archives of Internal Medicine* **138**: 969–73

Sin DD, Wu l, Anderson JA, et al. (2005) Inhaled corticosteroids and mortality in chronic obstructive pulmonary disease. *Thorax* **60**: 992–7

Sutherland ER, Allmers H, Ayas NT, et al. (2003) Inhaled corticosteroids reduce the progression of airflow obstruction in COPD; a meta-analysis. *Thorax* **58**: 937–41

Van Grunsven PM, van Schayck CP, Derenne JP, et al. (1999) Long term effects of inhaled corticosteroids in chronic obstructive pulmonary disease: a meta-analysis. *Thorax* **54**: 7–14

COMBINED LONG-ACTING BRONCHODILATORS AND INHALED CORTICOSTEROIDS

Main points

1 Adding a long-acting beta-agonist and inhaled corticosteroid in a combined inhaler achieves better outcomes than either drug alone.

2 There is evidence that triple therapy with a LABA, LAMA and inhaled corticosteroid may have further benefits in some patients and has been endorsed by NICE.

3 The recent TORCH study suggests that combined salmeterol/fluticasone combination may have an effect on reducing mortality (all cause mortality reduced by 17% compared with placebo) but the data just failed to reach statistical significance.

Since 2002 there have been a series of large, important trials, which have considerably improved our knowledge of therapy in COPD and have provided the evidence base for effective management of COPD patients. Combined therapy has been shown since the mid-1990s to be highly effective in controlling asthma. All the studies in COPD have shown significant improvements in lung function, symptoms and quality of life, and reduction in exacerbations.

Since the introduction of tiotropium, studies looking at various combinations of triple therapy (LABA, LAMA and inhaled corticosteroid) have been performed, with suggestions of greater improvement in lung function but less clear-cut benefits in other clinical parameters. NICE has endorsed using all three groups of therapy in more severely symptomatic patients.

Salmeterol/fluticasone studies

Mahler et al. (2002) carried out a 6-month four-arm study with placebo, salmeterol, fluticasone 500 µg twice daily and a combination of active drugs. All active treatments produced improvements in lung function and breathlessness, and a reduction in reliever therapy, but the combined drug achieved significantly greater change than either drug alone.

The TRISTAN study – the Trial of Inhaled Steroids and Long-Acting Beta-2 Agonists (Calverley et al. 2003a) – used the same design but was for one year and looked at other clinical outcomes. Lung function and symptom improvements mirrored those found by Mahler. In addition, the combined agent, but not the single drugs on their own, achieved a clinically meaningful improvement in health status greater than 4 points (St George's Respiratory Questionnaire; SGRQ) and a reduction in exacerbations, particularly in patients with more severe disease and an FEV_1 below 50% predicted.

The TORCH study (Towards a Revolution in COPD Health) (2008) was a large, randomised trial of 6112 patients comparing, in a four-arm study, salmeterol/fluticasone combination, the component drugs on their own and placebo, over a follow-up period of 3 years. The primary outcome was all cause mortality with exacerbations, health status and lung function also being assessed.

Mortality was reduced by 17% in the combined arm, but this just failed to hit statistical significance, p = 0.052. The causes of death were well documented and there were high proportions due to cardiovascular disease and cancer as well as respiratory causes (see Figure 3.1). For the other outcomes the combination therapy showed a 25% reduction in exacerbations (less for single therapies), and a 17% reduction in hospital admissions. The combined therapy produced a 3.1 unit change in SGRQ score over 3 years and an improvement in FEV_1 of 92ml compared with placebo. The main adverse effect was the previously mentioned increase in pneumonia in the corticosteroid containing arms of the trial.

A further analysis of TORCH data on rate of decline in FEV_1 showed rates of 55ml/year for placebo, 42ml/year for both salmeterol and fluticasone on their own and 39ml/year for the combination – a difference that was significant. This suggests combined therapy slows disease progression. This is perhaps due to the reduction in exacerbation frequency, as we know that frequent exacerbations are associated with a more rapid decline in lung function.

Formoterol/budesonide studies

A one-year study by Szafranski et al. (2003), with a similar four-arm design to the salmeterol/fluticasone studies, used budesonide in the lower dose of 800µg per day in the combined and single inhaler. There were similar significant improvements for all active treatments, with greater lung function, reduced symptoms and an almost clinically significant change of 3.9 points on the SGRQ health status score. Exacerbations were reduced by 24% using the combined drug compared with placebo.

A further study by Calverley et al. (2003a, b) had a slightly different design: patients were given two weeks of prednisolone initially and then followed up for one year. Lung function with the combined therapy maintained the prednisolone-induced improvement while all other therapies declined towards baseline. The combined treatment further enhanced the improvement in the SGRQ score from 4 to 7 points with only mild deterioration in other active treatments. A reduction in exacerbation rate similar to that in the previous study was noted.

The results from these studies show very consistent findings which are most beneficial to patients. The NICE update suggests combined therapy should effectively be offered to any patient with persisting symptoms who is having regular exacerbations, irrespective of level of FEV_1 percent predicted.

Triple therapy

There have been few trials that compare three drugs against their components apart from one physiological study which showed superior lung function for three drugs. A study called INSPIRE compared salmeterol/fluticasone with tiotropium with no differences found in exacerbation frequency and a slight benefit of the combination in health status. Considerable numbers of patients dropped out of the study before completion, which makes interpretation difficult (Cochrane review).

A study adding formotrol/budesonide to tiotropium – that is comparing one drug against three – showed improved lung function and health status and less exacerbations for the three drugs, which is hardly surprising.

Further reading

Calverley P, Pauwels R, Vestbo J, et al. (2003a) Combined salmeterol and fluticasone in the treatment of chronic obstructive pulmonary disease: a randomised controlled trial (TRISTAN). *Lancet* **361**: 449–56

Calverley PM, Boonsawat W, Cseke Z, et al. (2003b) Maintenance therapy with budesonide and formoterol in COPD. *European Respiratory Journal* **22**: 912–19

Calverley P, Anderson JA, Celli B, et al. (2008) Salmeterol and fluticasone propionate and survival in chronic obstructive pulmonary disease. The TORCH study. *New England Journal of Medicine* **356**: 775–89

Celli B, Thomas NE, Anderson JA, et al. (2008) Effect of pharmacotherapy on rate of decline of lung function in obstructive pulmonary disease. Results from the TORCH study. *American Journal of Respiratory and Critical Care Medicine* **178**: 332–8

Mahler DA, Wire P, Horstman D, et al. (2002) Effectiveness of fluticasone and salmeterol combination delivered by the Diskus device in the treatment of COPD. *American Journal of Respiratory and Critical Care Medicine* **166**: 1084–91

Szafranski W, Cukier A, Ramirez G et al. (2003) Efficacy and safety of budesonide/formoterol in the management of COPD. *European Respiratory Journal* **21**: 74–81

Wedzicha JA, Calverly PMA, Seemungal T, et al. (2008) The prevention of chronic obstructive pulmonary disease exacerbations by salmeterol/fluticasone propionate or tiotropium bromide. (INSPIRE study). *American Journal of Respiratory and Critical Care Medicine* **177**: 19–26

MUCOLYTICS

Mucolytics, such as carbocisteine and mecysteine, have a role in the management of COPD, particularly for patients with chronic bronchitis. They can be used in two ways.

1 To make sputum less sticky and more fluid, thus making it easier for patients with chronic bronchitis to clear sputum if their cough is troublesome and having an adverse effect on quality of life. It is not suitable for those patients who do not have a persistent cough or who have a cough with watery sputum.

2   To reduce the frequency of exacerbations, particularly in patients who are not taking inhaled corticosteroids.

Mucolytics are an oral medication and, when used to improve the quality of coughing, should be given as a trial of therapy for 4–6 weeks. Assessment of success is on patient questioning. Used in this way therapy may be used over the winter months or more continuously.

When mucolytics are used to prevent exacerbations, the choice of patient should include those who have at least two exacerbations per year and particularly those who are not taking or are intolerant of an inhaled corticosteroid. If mucolytics show benefit they should be used long term. The NICE update stipulates that mucolytics should not be used routinely for this indication. However, a recent Cochrane review (2010) has shown a 21% reduction in exacerbations and also a decrease in the total days of disability.

A new mucolytic called erdosteine is licenced for use only during exacerbations and should be prescribed for only 10 days.

Further reading

Poole P, Black PN (2010) Mucolytic agents for chronic bronchitis or chronic obstructive pulmonary disease. *Cochrane database of Systematic Reviews 2010*: **Issue 2**.
Rudolf M, Bellamy D, Burrill P, et al. (2010) Consensus guideline for the prolonged use of mucolytic therapy in patients with diagnosed COPD. Guidelines **42**:119–22.

DRUG THERAPY OF THE FUTURE

Main points

1   Pharmaceutical companies are very active in the field of new therapies for COPD and many potential new drugs are under trial. New combinations of two or even three agents and once daily long-acting inhaled bronchodilators, such as the newly launched indacterol, are being investigated. Many of these look to be more effective than existing therapies

2   The first of the selective phosphodiesterase inhibitors –
    PDE4 inhibitors – roflumilast has been launched as a tablet
    and it is likely other products will follow.
3   The role of antioxidant therapy is being investigated, as are
    other anti-inflammatory therapies.

New inhaled long-acting bronchodilators and corticosteroids

Many pharmaceutical companies are trialling both long-acting beta-
agonists and anti-muscarinic agents as they are key to improving
symptoms and reducing the frequency of exacerbations. They are
also likely to be used for asthma. 2010 saw the launch of indacterol,
a once daily LABA, which has trial results as least as good as salmeterol and formoterol. Under development are carmoterol and
milveterol, as well as other unnamed agents that appear to have
good efficacy and safety profiles.

Likewise, there are a handful of LAMA drugs that will compete
with tiotropium.

Pharmaceutical companies are also testing new combination inhalers such as indacterol/mometasone or LABA/LAMA
combinations.

New once daily inhaled corticosteroid compounds are quite well
advanced and are likely to be available on their own for asthma and
in combination with a LABA for COPD and asthma.

Even triple therapy inhalers are likely.

Anti-inflammatory therapies

Increasingly, the design of new drugs is geared towards the pathological changes that are observed in disease processes. Inflammatory
changes are found in the airways of people with chronic bronchitis
and, to some extent, the terminal airways of patients with emphysema. There are increases in the number of inflammatory cells, such
as neutrophils, T-lymphocytes and alveolar macrophages.

Corticosteroids have a modest effect, so other means of blocking
the inflammatory process are being explored.

Leukotriene antagonists have had a beneficial role in asthma. There have, as yet, been no trials of these agents in COPD but it is unlikely that the currently available drugs that block the leukotriene receptors will have a major role. However, leukotriene LTB4 is a potent stimulator of neutrophils, and its levels are increased in the sputum of COPD patients. Trials are currently in progress with selective LTB4 inhibitors, which may be useful in reducing sputum production and cough in COPD.

Phosphodiesterase-4 (PDE4) inhibitors

The new oral once daily PDE4 inhibitor, roflumilast has recently been launched and is discussed in more detail earlier in this chapter. Other drugs in this new therapeutic group are under investigation. Studies are at a relatively early stage but PDE4 inhibitors act both as a bronchodilator, reducing symptoms, and to reduce exacerbation frequency. More comparative studies with existing forms of therapy are awaited.

Antiproteases

There is evidence to suggest that one of the major factors in the development of lung damage and emphysema in COPD is over-activity of proteolytic enzymes released from neutrophils and macrophages. The enhanced cellular breakdown may be related to more enzyme release or decreased protective mechanisms, as in alpha-1 antitrypsin deficiency. Neutrophil elastase inhibitors have been developed but are awaiting clinical trials.

Alpha-1 antitrypsin

The genetically inherited homozygous deficiency of the antiprotease protein alpha-1 antitrypsin leads to the development of emphysema in the third decade of life. Various clinical trials have attempted to replace alpha-1 antitrypsin but the results have generally been disappointing. Alpha-1 antitrypsin can be extracted from plasma but the cost is high. A trial in the USA using weekly intravenous alpha-1 antitrypsin failed to halt the decline in lung function. A nebulised formulation – also very expensive – has been tried but, again, improvements are minimal.

Antioxidants

There is good evidence that active oxygen radicals, present in cigarette smoke, play an important role in damaging the lungs in COPD. They are also released by inflammatory cells such as neutrophils and macrophages. The results of a number of studies have suggested that diets high in fresh fruit and vegetables, which contain many antioxidants, may help to prevent or slow the rate of progress of COPD as well as having favourable effects on various cancers, heart disease and bowel disease.

N-Acetyl cysteine

This drug started life as a mucolytic agent but had only mild clinical effects on sputum. However, it also has antioxidant properties and a Cochrane review has revealed that it does have beneficial actions in COPD. The results of a meta-analysis against placebo showed a 29% reduction in exacerbations, and those in the group receiving treatment had fewer days of illness. There was no difference in lung function or in adverse events between treatments. In a separate, uncontrolled, study there was a reduction in the rate of decline in FEV_1.

N-Acetyl cysteine is not licensed for use in the UK.

Statins

Statins have been shown to have anti-inflammatory and immune modulating effects. There have been a number of positive trials thus far showing reduced COPD exacerbations, improved lung function and exercise capability, and reduced all cause mortality. Their role in long-term COPD management has yet to be established.

Drugs for pulmonary hypertension

Pulmonary hypertension is a serious complication of severe COPD which increases symptoms and worsens prognosis. It is difficult to study such patients and trial patient numbers are thus small. Various groups of drugs have been and continue to be assessed but there have been few clinically positive results.

Vasodilators such as those used in systemic hypertension have no real effect. Phosphodiesterase 5 inhibitors such as sildenafil may help in other forms of pulmonary hypertension but not significantly in COPD. Endothelial receptor antagonists dilate pulmonary vessels but have no worthwhile benefit in COPD. Prostaglandins are being investigated as are statins.

Further reading

Barnes PJ, Stockley RA (2005) COPD; current therapeutic interventions and future approaches. *European Respiratory Journal* **25**: 1084–106

Cazzola M, Matera MG (2009) Emerging inhaled bronchodilators; an update. *European Respiratory Journal* **34**: 757–69

Decramer M, Janssens W (2010) Mucoactive therapy in COPD. *European Respiratory Review* **19**: 134–40

Janda S, Park K, Fitzgerald M, et al (2009) Statins in COPD. A systematic review. *Chest* **136**: 734–43

9 | Pulmonary rehabilitation

Main points

1 Pulmonary rehabilitation has been shown to produce clinically and statistically significant improvements in:
   - health-related quality of life
   - functional and maximal exercise capacity
   - breathlessness.
   The magnitude of these effects is greater than that produced by bronchodilator therapy.

2 Pulmonary rehabilitation may also lead to a reduction in hospital admissions and in-patient stays.

3 There is good evidence that out-patient pulmonary rehabilitation is both effective and cost effective in COPD.

4 Rehabilitation should be available to *all* patients who feel they are functionally disabled by their COPD – a score of 3 or more on the MRC dyspnoea scale – including those who have had a recent hospitalisation for an exacerbation.

5 The cornerstone of rehabilitation is individually prescribed exercise endurance training.

6 Exercise for specific muscle groups can improve functional ability and may be particularly useful for patients with very severe disease.

7 Education about the disease and its management, nutrition, relaxation and coping strategies, and the management of exacerbations should also be included.

8 The patient's carer should be actively encouraged to be involved in the rehabilitation programme.

9 Support and encouragement to continue with lifestyle changes at the end of the programme are helpful.

10 *All patients benefit from keeping active.* Patients, in all healthcare settings, should be encouraged to maintain, and preferably increase, their activity levels.

Pulmonary rehabilitation is an increasingly popular and effective intervention for people with moderate and severe COPD. Historically, management focused on strategies either to prevent deterioration (stopping smoking) or to improve lung function (using bronchodilators and corticosteroids). Treatment that aimed to improve quality of life or health status and functional ability received little attention. The nature of COPD – *fixed or partially fixed airflow obstruction* – means that improvement in lung function (impairment) can be at best modest, whereas improvement in patients' functional performance and health status (disability and handicap) can be considerable. Pulmonary rehabilitation focuses on these areas.

Evidence for the effectiveness of rehabilitation in COPD

A dictionary definition of rehabilitation is:

'to restore to good condition; to make fit after disablement or illness.'

Rehabilitation aims to restore the individual to the best physical, mental and emotional state possible. The ethos of rehabilitation has been embraced enthusiastically in the fields of cardiology, orthopaedics and neurology. In the UK, however, it has been adopted only slowly in respiratory medicine even though all the national and international COPD guidelines state that rehabilitation is an important part of COPD management. The 2004 NICE guideline stated that rehabilitation should be offered and available to any COPD patient who feels they are disabled by their condition, so it is disappointing that the provision of pulmonary rehabilitation in the UK, whilst it has improved, is still 'patchy'. The National Clinical Strategy strongly supports rehabilitation, so it is hoped that access will continue to improve in future.

Whether pulmonary rehabilitation has an effect on mortality from COPD is not proven. It seems that the most important factor in determining survival is the post-bronchodilator FEV_1. However, maximal exercise capacity is also a factor in determining prognosis, and it is therefore logical to suppose that pulmonary rehabilitation, that improves maximal exercise capacity, may also have a beneficial effect on mortality. It must be borne in mind, though, that extending the life of a COPD patient is not the prime aim of rehabilitation. Rather, it is to improve the quality and reduce the dependence of their remaining years.

There is plenty of evidence that pulmonary rehabilitation is effective in reducing breathlessness and improving exercise tolerance. Controlled studies have revealed that the sensation of dyspnoea is reduced and exercise capacity is increased after exercise training. Health-related quality of life scores also improve following rehabilitation programmes.

Evidence from the USA has shown that pulmonary rehabilitation reduces the need for health care. There, programmes are sometimes eligible for reimbursement by insurers because they have been found to substantially reduce both hospital admission rates and inpatient stays. Unscheduled, emergency care is a major cost in the UK and there is now considerable pressure to reduce both the number of admissions and the length of stay. The evidence from UK studies that pulmonary rehabilitation can contribute to this is controversial. Whilst some observational, non-randomised studies have demonstrated reduced admissions and in-patient stays, others have not found a significant advantage over usual care. Obviously, the financial saving to the health service depends on the cost of the rehabilitation programme, but they are generally 'low tech' and cheap compared with the cost of admitting a patient to hospital because of an exacerbation of COPD.

Health economic data from UK centres has confirmed that pulmonary rehabilitation is cost effective. Even when all indirect costs such as transport and carers' time off work have been taken into consideration, it costs no more to rehabilitate COPD patients than to treat them without rehabilitation.

Why rehabilitation programmes are needed

Breathlessness on exertion and the fear, anxiety and panic it engenders often lead a person with COPD to avoid activity. Attacks of breathlessness or coughing that occur outside the home may cause particular anxiety and embarrassment. Exercise avoidance results in deconditioning of skeletal muscles, and contributes to the loss of muscle mass that occurs as a result of systemic inflammatory processes in COPD. This increases disability; COPD patients often report that the limiting factor to their exercise tolerance is tiredness in the legs rather than breathlessness. Avoiding exercise, as well as the fear that breathlessness invokes, leads to a general loss of confidence, sowing the seeds of social isolation and increasing dependence. Increasing inactivity and isolation further compound the problem and the patient is in a vicious circle that results in increasing dependence, disability and worsening quality of life (Figure 9.1.)

For many COPD patients the 'normal' irritations and stresses of everyday life are sufficient to induce breathlessness. The phenomenon of the 'emotional straitjacket' of advanced COPD is widely recognised.

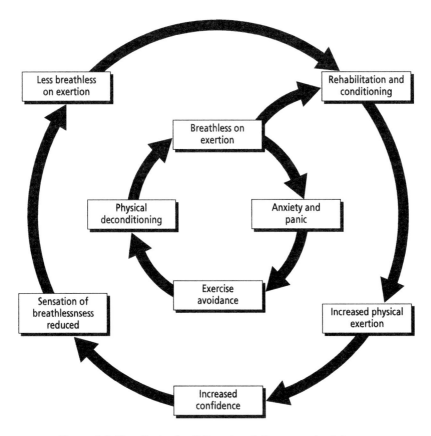

Figure 9.1 The affects of activity or inactivity on exercise tolerance
(Reproduced by permission of Education for Health)

- A passive dependent role may be adopted, in which the patient takes little part in family life.

- Patients feel they are a burden to their families.

- Frustration is often expressed as anger, usually directed at the family carer.

- Guilt at what is seen as a 'self-inflicted' disease is another common emotion.

- Resentment on the part of the carer at the restrictions this disease imposes on long-held plans for retirement may also be manifest.

- Self-destructive patterns of behaviour, such as a refusal to contemplate stopping smoking, are often seen.

- Self-esteem is frequently very low, and depression is common.

- Many patients refuse to exercise or will be restrained by an over-protective carer from exercising, even within their limited potential.

The aim of pulmonary rehabilitation is to break this vicious circle of increasing inactivity and breathlessness and to improve exercise capacity and functional ability.

The setting and timing of pulmonary rehabilitation

Pulmonary rehabilitation has traditionally taken place as a hospital out-patient programme. Some centres also offer inpatient rehabilitation and in some areas home or primary-care-based programmes are available. An encouraging development in recent years has been the increase in the number of community-based programmes.

The majority of studies have been conducted in the out-patient setting and, as yet there is limited evidence for the effectiveness of community-based programmes and a lack of comparative studies. However, community-based programmes are likely to be more accessible and, provided they adhere to current guidelines regarding course content, duration, patient assessment, exercise prescription, and staffing, there is no reason to suppose that they would be any less effective than hospital-based rehabilitation.

Perhaps the most important factors for increasing access and improving adherence to pulmonary rehabilitation programmes is to ensure that rehabilitation occurs:

- in places with good access for people with respiratory disability (there is adequate parking close by and, if necessary, a lift)
- at times that suit patients
- within a reasonable time of referral.

The NICE update (2010) examined the timing of pulmonary rehabilitation, and specifically the efficacy of rehabilitation commenced within a month of a hospitalisation for an exacerbation of COPD. In some of the studies examined rehabilitation commenced in hospital and the patient joined an out-patient programme on discharge. Despite some problems with methodology and data analysis NICE note that the existing studies suggest that there is some benefit to early rehabilitation and recommend that patients should not be excluded from referral if they have had a recent exacerbation.

The components of pulmonary rehabilitation

Pulmonary rehabilitation programmes consist of three main components:

- exercise training
- education about the disease and its management
- psychosocial support.

Exercise

Exercise (aerobic) training to recondition skeletal muscles and improve exercise endurance forms the cornerstone of most programmes. The amount of exercise prescribed is determined on an individual basis and is based either on a laboratory treadmill or cycle ergometer test or a field exercise test, such as the relatively simple incremental shuttle walking test (see Chapter 6). The shuttle walking test is closely related to an individual's peak oxygen consumption (VO_2 peak) and allows a reasonably accurate prescription of exercise. It has been suggested that, when there is no access to exercise-testing equipment, patients may be able to determine their own training regimen, based on their perception of breathlessness. A Borg scale (see Table 6.4) is often employed, and the patient is encouraged to exercise to between levels 3 and 5 (moderate to severe).

Most programmes use cycling or walking for exercise endurance training. Generally, an attempt is made to prescribe a form of regular exercise that the patient will find easy to continue at home both during and after the rehabilitation programme. Walking and cycling are also activities that have some meaning for the patient in terms of their daily lives.

Exercises that train specific groups of muscles are included in a training programme. Lower limb exercises improve exercise tolerance while upper limb exercises improve the patient's ability to perform particular tasks associated with daily living. In someone with COPD the accessory muscles of respiration may be used. Any activity that uses the same muscle groups, such as brushing the hair or carrying shopping, is likely to increase the breathlessness. Specific exercises for particular muscle groups may be of great benefit for patients with severe COPD, who may find aerobic exercise too demanding. The exercises are generally of the more gentle bend-and-stretch variety, but may still give good results in increasing functional ability.

The benefit of respiratory muscle training as part of a pulmonary rehabilitation programme is not proven and it is not recommended as a routine. Training the respiratory muscles for strength and endurance has been successful in healthy subjects and in patients with chronic airflow obstruction but evidence that such training produces clinically significant results in patients with COPD is lacking.

Hospital-based pulmonary rehabilitation programmes are generally multidisciplinary and do not consist of exercise training alone. The first hour of a session is usually devoted to an exercise routine and the second hour to educating the patient and family about the disease, its management and how to develop strategies to live with it (summarised in Table 9.1). Partners and carers are generally actively encouraged to attend. A carer's need for information and social support is often as great as, if not greater than, the patient's.

Table 9.1 Components of pulmonary rehabilitation

Exercise
Endurance (aerobic) training:
  Walking
  Cycling
Specific muscle groups (e.g. upper limb girdle)
?Respiratory muscle training (value debatable)

Education
The lungs in health and disease
Drug treatment
Self-management
Stopping smoking
Nutrition
Breathing control and sputum clearance
Relaxation techniques/coping strategies
Dealing with everyday activities
Financial support and benefits
(Some centres also discuss 'end of life planning' and
  palliative care with appropriate groups)

Education and advice

People need basic information about the lungs in health and disease to help them understand the role of smoking in the development of COPD. Some centres exclude patients who continue to smoke but others will accept them and include smoking cessation in their education programme. Studies of people who fail to complete a rehabilitation programme have, however, identified continuing smokers as being less likely to successfully complete a programme. Other groups less likely to complete are those who are widowed or divorced, live alone or have poor levels of social support. There is certainly some logic to accepting smokers for rehabilitation. If they are excluded, a low self-esteem – 'I'm not worth the trouble' – may well be reinforced. Joining a programme with other COPD sufferers who have successfully 'kicked the habit' may provide added incentive for an attempt to quit. However, when resources are strained offering places to those most likely to complete the course and gain the most benefit is also a logical, if not strictly equitable approach. It should be born in mind that NICE have stated that there is,

> *'...currently no justification for selection on the basis of age, impairment, disability, smoking status or use of oxygen. The only issues material to selection are poor motivation and the logistical factors of geography, transport, equipment usage, and the group composition.'*

Advice is also given about the drug treatment of COPD and how to manage exacerbations effectively. Other professionals may be involved in giving additional education. For example:

- Dieticians can provide valuable general advice on healthy eating; they are also available to provide specific advice to the overweight or underweight patient.

- A physiotherapist can teach sputum clearance techniques and breathing control. Relaxation and coping skills are also valuable.

- The occupational therapist can provide advice or equipment to help with activities of daily living.

- The social worker may be able to give advice on benefits and financial matters.

Marital and sexual problems are common among these patients, so specialist help and advice may also be needed. The personnel involved varies widely, depending very much on local circumstances.

Psychosocial support

Many patients with advanced COPD are socially isolated. Pulmonary rehabilitation programmes can provide both patients and their partners/carers with valuable social contact. The support provided by group members can be enormous.

A pulmonary rehabilitation programme should consist of two or three supervised, group sessions a week for 6–12 weeks, combined with a programme of exercises the patient performs at home between sessions. Unsupervised exercise programmes can produce improvements in breathlessness, but are not as effective as supervised, group sessions.

The improvement gained in a rehabilitation programme decreases over time and, to date, there is limited evidence that repeat programmes confer additional benefit. The provision of follow-up and after-care would probably be beneficial, but this is an area that needs further, high-quality research. Clearly, for after-care to be provided indefinitely in a hospital setting would be expensive and, it could be argued, might serve to undermine the philosophy of self-reliance that is engendered as part of the initial programme.

The provision of a 'training diary' or an occasional 'refresher' session is offered by some centres as a solution to the problem of continuing support. In others, patients 'graduate' from pulmonary rehabilitation to a patient support group. The British Lung Foundation's Breathe Easy groups provide an ideal forum for continuing social contact, support and encouragement. Some centres graduate less severely disabled patients to an 'exercise on prescription' group at local sports centres where they can still meet regularly, exercise and benefit from mutual support (see end of chapter for address).

The role of the primary health care team

The role of the primary health care team is:

- to select appropriate patients for referral

- to support and encourage patients undergoing rehabilitation

- to follow-up and provide continued encouragement for patients who have graduated from hospital programmes.

Before a referral for rehabilitation is considered, it should be ensured that the patient is on optimum therapy and that no further improvements with additional drug intervention can be achieved. It is also important to consider whether the patient's disability is related solely to COPD or if there is a significant co-morbidity that will limit the effectiveness of rehabilitation. For example, a patient who has severe rheumatoid arthritis or ischaemic heart disease may be unable to undertake the exercise component of the programme. Some centres will accept such patients for the education component of the programme, but they are unlikely to gain the same degree of benefit.

The selection of appropriate patients is crucial and is not based solely on clinical criteria (Table 9.2):

- Current smokers might not be accepted, as discussed earlier. Some physicians consider that patients who are unable to stop smoking are unlikely to be able to make the lifestyle changes that are at the core of rehabilitation and are also unlikely to adhere to an exercise programme.

- Difficulties with travel may mean that ambulance transport will have to be arranged.

- If the patient is still working, there may be difficulties with attending all the sessions.

- Perhaps the most important consideration of all is *the patient's motivation to improve*. Patients need to be informed of the benefits, but also need to understand the commitment they must make in order to gain them.

Table 9.2 Patient selection

Motivated to improve
On optimal treatment and compliant with treatment
Increasing disability
Able to exercise (caution with cardiac, orthopaedic or neurological problems)

If your area includes people from ethnic minorities, there may be language and culture difficulties. However, it may be possible to gather a group of patients of the same ethnic origin and use an interpreter who can also advise on cultural aspects.

The fact that a patient is using oxygen is not a reason to exclude them from a rehabilitation programme, and neither is the severity of their condition. It could be argued that patients with severe disease stand to gain the most from rehabilitation.

Where there are currently no formal rehabilitation programmes, and for those patients who are unable or decline to attend, the primary health care team may need to be innovative and enlist whatever services are available locally. Protected time in a structured COPD clinic in general practice can provide a useful forum for delivering basic education about COPD to patients and their carers. A community physiotherapist, particularly if they have a respiratory interest, may be a useful resource. Leaflets containing information about suitable gentle exercises and breathing control are available from the British Lung Foundation (see the 'Useful address' at the end of this chapter). Patients need to be reassured that getting breathless when exercising will not cause any further damage to their lungs, and they should all be encouraged to keep active, maintaining, and preferably improving, their activity level by taking some form of regular exercise. A daily walk or regular stair climbing fits well with everyday life and may be more likely to be adhered to on a regular basis than a series of exercises that the patient sees as bearing little relation to their normal activities.

Rehabilitation may be unfamiliar territory for the primary care team. When advising about exercise there can be understandable concerns if the patient also suffers from ischaemic heart disease.

It may be better, therefore, to start with an 'uncomplicated' patient and to keep advice simple and practical. Giving your patients the following cycle of exercises can be a useful starting point.

The family focus of primary care and its ability to provide long-term follow-up and care make it an ideal setting for the education, follow-up and encouragement of COPD patients and their families.

Finally, when you are encouraging someone to exercise, the type is perhaps less important than its regularity. It is important not to deter patients with too rigid or complicated an exercise regimen. The essence is to encourage, to reassure that they will do themselves no harm and, perhaps most important of all, to persuade them that they are worth the effort.

Further reading

Bestall JC, Paul EA, Garrod R, et al. (2003) Longitudinal trends in exercise capacity and health status after pulmonary rehabilitation in patients with COPD. *Respiratory Medicine* **97**(2): 173–80

British Thoracic Society Standards of Care Subcommittee on Pulmonary Rehabilitation. (2001) Pulmonary rehabilitation. *Thorax* **56**(11): 827–34

Griffiths TL, Phillips CJ, Davies S, Burr ML, Campbell IA (2001) Cost effectiveness of an outpatient multidisciplinary pulmonary rehabilitation programme. *Thorax* **56**: 779–84

Lacasse Y, Brosseau L, Milne S, et al. (2003) Pulmonary rehabilitation for chronic obstructive pulmonary disease. *The Cochrane Library*; **3**(3)

Morgan M, Singh S (1997) *Practical Pulmonary Rehabilitation.* Chapman and Hall Medical, London.

National Clinical Guideline Centre (2010) Chronic obstructive pulmonary disease: the management of chronic obstructive pulmonary disease in adults in primary and secondary care. London. CG101. Available at http://guidance.nice.org.uk/CG101/Guidance/pdf/English.

Useful address

Breathe Easy Club
British Lung Foundation
73–75 Goswell Road
London EC1V 7ER
Tel: 020 7688 5555
Fax: 020 7688 5556
Website: www.lunguk.org

(Exercise instructions and drawings on pages 162–165 reproduced by permission of Education for Health.)

1 Shoulder shrugging.
Circle your shoulder forwards, down, backwards and up. Keep the timing constant, allowing two full seconds per circle and relax throughout. Continue for 30 seconds. Repeat the exercise three times with short rests in between.

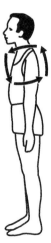

2 Full arm circling.
One arm at a time, pass your arm as near as possible to the side of your head; move your arm in as large a circle as possible (10 seconds per circle). Repeat for 40 seconds. Repeat the exercise three times with short rests in between. Do the same now with the other arm.

3 Increasing arm circles.

Hold one arm away from your body at shoulder height. Progressively increase the size of the circle for a count of six circles in 10 seconds, then decrease it over a further count of six. Repeat for 40 seconds. Do the same now with the other arm.

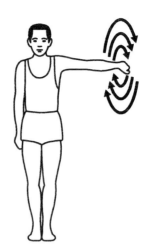

4 Abdominal exercises.

Sitting in chair, tighten your abdominal muscles, hold for a count of four and then release the muscles over four seconds to the starting position. Repeat continuously for 30 seconds. Do the procedure three times with short rests in between.

5 Wall press-ups.

Stand with your feet a full arm's length away from the wall, place your hands on wall and bend at the elbows until your nose touches the wall. Push your arms straight again, allowing eight seconds from start to completion. Repeat for 40 seconds continuously to a total of five repetitions. Repeat the procedure three times with short rests in between.

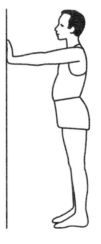
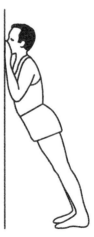

6 Sitting to standing.
Using an ordinary chair, sit, stand and sit, allowing 10 seconds from start to completion. Repeat continuously for 40 seconds to a total of five repetitions. Do the exercise three times with short rests in between.

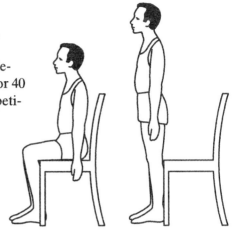

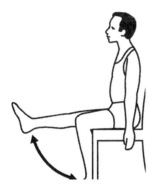

7 Quadriceps exercise.
Sitting on an ordinary chair, straighten your right knee and tense your thigh muscles; hold for a count of four, then relax gradually over a further four seconds. Do this a total of five repetitions over 40 seconds. Repeat the exercise three times with short rest periods in between. Do the same now with your left leg.

8 Calf exercises.
Holding onto the back of a chair, go up on your toes and then back, taking 8–10 seconds to complete procedure. Repeat this continuously for 40 seconds.

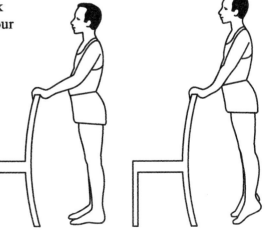

9 Walking on the spot.

Holding onto the back of a chair, allow one knee to bend, keeping your toes on the ground. Bend the other knee while straightening the first knee, allowing four seconds for the complete procedure. Repeat this bending and straightening of your knees (i.e.walking on the spot), keeping your toes on the ground, continuously for 40 seconds – a total of 10 times. Repeat the exercise three times with short rest periods in between.

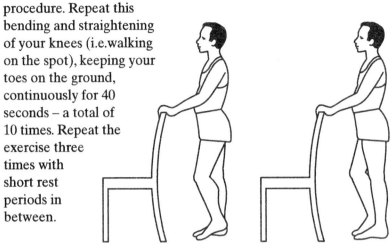

10 Step-ups.

Step up with your right foot onto step then bring up your left foot. Step down with your right foot and then your left foot. Allow four seconds for the complete procedure and repeat continuously for 40 seconds – a total of 10 times. Repeat the exercise three times with short rest periods between.

10 | Other forms of therapy

Main points

Oxygen

1   As COPD progresses patients may develop chronic hypoxia, which shortens life expectancy. Long-term oxygen therapy (LTOT) in these patients improves survival as well as reducing the incidence of polycythaemia and the progression of pulmonary hypertension.

2   The need for LTOT should be assessed in **all** patients with very severe COPD (FEV_1 less than 30% predicted) and in those with less severe disease (FEV_1 30–49% predicted) if there is evidence of:

- cyanosis
- peripheral oedema
- raised jugular venous pressure
- polycythaemia
- oxygen saturation 92% or less breathing air.

In order that all patients eligible for LTOT are identified, pulse oximeters should be available in all healthcare settings and saturations routinely measured in all COPD patients with moderate and severe disease.

3   To be effective, LTOT must be administered for at least 15 hours per day, and longer than this produces greater benefit.

4   The most cost-effective way of administering oxygen over long periods is by oxygen concentrator.

5   Ambulatory oxygen systems are now available for those patients using LTOT who are able and wish to use oxygen outside the home.

6   A few patients with COPD desaturate on exercise. Ambulatory oxygen may prevent desaturation and improve

exercise tolerance and breathlessness, but should only be prescribed after thorough, specialist assessment.

7 Short-burst oxygen therapy is expensive and of unproven benefit in COPD. It should only be prescribed as part of palliative care or for patients who remain breathless despite other therapy.

8 Inappropriate oxygen therapy in COPD patients can suppress respiratory drive and worsen respiratory failure. Particular care is needed with administration of oxygen in exacerbations and in transit to hospital.

9 Some patients on LTOT who are chronically hypercapnic, or who have needed ventilation during an exacerbation may benefit from non-invasive ventilation at home

10 Patients with severe COPD need specialist advice before flying or travelling to high altitude.

Surgery

1 The surgical removal of large bullae may significantly improve lung function and symptoms.

2 Surgery to reduce lung volume is gaining in popularity but should be performed only in specialist centres and with careful patient selection. It has an operative mortality of 1–3% but can produce good clinical improvements.

3 Lung transplants are usually performed on younger patients (below 50 years) with alpha-1 antitrypsin deficiency emphysema.

Vaccination and antiviral drugs

1 Annual vaccination against influenza is recommended and should be actively encouraged in COPD patients.

2 The Department of Health recommends pneumococcal vaccination for patients with COPD.

3 The antiviral drugs, oseltamivir and zanamivir are recommended for the treatment of influenza and, in some circumstances for post-exposure prophylaxis in patients who are not adequately protected by influenza vaccination.

Nutrition

1   Diets rich in antioxidants (e.g. fresh fruit and vegetables) may help to slow the progress of COPD.

2   Obese patients should be vigorously encouraged to lose weight, which will reduce breathlessness and improve mobility.

3   Many patients with advanced emphysema are underweight and have extensive muscle wasting. The mechanism is not certain but inflammatory cytokines may have a role.

4   Patients with muscle wasting need advice on an appropriate diet.

5   Life expectancy is worse for COPD patients who are underweight and have muscle wasting.

Oxygen therapy

Patients with severe COPD who are in chronic respiratory failure benefit from oxygen, but it has to be given over long periods every day. The aims of long-term oxygen therapy (LTOT) are thus quite different from the short-term use of oxygen in hospital for patients with acute exacerbations.

At sea level the atmosphere contains around 21% oxygen. LTOT aims to increase the concentration of oxygen in inhaled air to around 30%. This level generally provides the best tissue oxygenation without increasing the arterial carbon dioxide and worsening the respiratory failure. The results of two placebo-controlled trials of LTOT revealed:

* improved survival

* reduced polycythaemia

* no progression of pulmonary hypertension

* slightly improved health status.

The first of these trials, conducted by the Medical Research Council (MRC), showed that 15 hours of oxygen per day increased five-year survival from 25% to 41%. The second trial – the Nocturnal Oxygen

Therapy Trial (NOTT) – demonstrated that continuous oxygen (mean use of 17.7 hours per day) was beneficial, but that use for only 12 hours per day conferred no benefit.

A further study of patients using 15 hours of oxygen per day showed that, although five-year survival was 62%, this had dropped to only 26% at 10 years. Why some patients do better than others is incompletely understood. Generally, the patients who obtained most benefit from LTOT had:

- a higher $PaCO_2$
- a higher packed cell volume (haematocrit)
- a higher pulmonary pressure
- a lower FVC.

A good prognostic indicator was a fall in pulmonary artery pressure of more than 5mmHg over 24 hours when oxygen was given.

The clinical benefits of LTOT, apart from increased life expectancy, are an increase in exercise tolerance and reduced breathlessness. Whether LTOT improves health status is debatable. A striking finding in patients being considered for LTOT is the very high level of emotional and mood disturbance. These patients have severe disease: depression is thus very common and low self-esteem almost universal. Whilst the NOTT study did not show any change in health status on oxygen, the results from other studies have indicated improvement in mood and depression indices, well-being and breathlessness scores, exercise tolerance and sleep patterns. Generally, physicians with extensive experience of LTOT are favourably impressed with the improvements in quality of life that these patients can achieve.

Who should receive LTOT?

In general, patients considered for LTOT:

- have severe, and very severe COPD
- are hypoxic
- have evidence of right ventricular strain and peripheral oedema.

It is important to emphasise that patients being considered for LTOT must be assessed for this by a specialist. The oxygen flow rate that corrects the hypoxia without increasing carbon dioxide retention needs to be determined for the safe and effective administration of oxygen to these individuals. In some areas LTOT assessments are now undertaken in nurse-led services, or 'outreach' clinics.

Measurements of arterial blood gases are essential. If the criteria outlined below are met, the patient needs a trial of oxygen with further measurement of blood gases to determine what concentration of oxygen is required to correct the hypoxia without causing an undue increase in the level of carbon dioxide. It is essential that arterial blood gases for assessment for LTOT are taken when the patient has been clinically stable for at least a month. Drug therapy should be optimised and the possibility of further benefit from increased bronchodilator doses or improved delivery systems investigated.

Patients should have stopped smoking. Smoking, and naked flames in the presence of oxygen constitute a significant explosive hazard, which patients and their families need to be warned about. In addition, patients who smoke will continue to experience an accelerated decline in FEV_1 and reduced life-expectancy as a result. Although the evidence that LTOT has **no** benefit for continuing smokers is not conclusive, the 1999 Royal College of Physicians (RCP) Clinical Guideline for oxygen therapy, on which the NICE recommendations are based, suggests that it is inappropriate to prescribe LTOT to patients unwilling to stop smoking.

Although the decision to refer a patient for oxygen therapy is best made on clinical grounds together with the spirometry, pulse oximetry is a useful screening tool that should be universally available in general practice. If the oxygen saturation is less than 92% when the patient is stable, referral for blood gases and further investigation is indicated. NICE recommends that oxygen saturation be routinely measured in patients whose FEV_1 is less than 50% predicted.

Clinical criteria for LTOT

The following are the recommendations from the Royal College of Physicians of London Clinical Guidelines 1999.

- Patients must be assessed when clinically stable for at least one month.

- They must have been optimally medically managed prior to assessment.

- The Pao$_2$ should be less than 7.3 kPa or 55mmHg when breathing air. The level of the carbon dioxide tension can be normal or elevated and does not influence the need for LTOT prescription.

- LTOT can be prescribed when the PaO$_2$ is between 7.3 and 8.0kPa together with the presence of one of the following:

  - secondary polycythaemia or nocturnal hypoxaemia (defined as SaO$_2$ below 90% for at least 30% of the night)

  - peripheral oedema

  - evidence of pulmonary hypertension.

- LTOT is not recommended for a PaO$_2$ above 8kPa.

- LTOT can be used for palliation of dyspnoea in disabling dyspnoea of terminal disease.

Oxygen should correct the blood gases to an arterial oxygen tension (PaO$_2$) greater than 8kPa, without causing a rise in arterial carbon dioxide (PaCO$_2$) that significantly increases the level of respiratory failure.

To confer any benefit, LTOT must be used for at least 15 hours per day. The NOTT study showed better survival in patients who used oxygen for 20 hours a day and the 2010 NICE update stresses that the hours of use of LTOT should not be restricted. In the case of LTOT – the longer the better! The most convenient and economical method of achieving 15 hours or more a day is with an oxygen concentrator.

Patients using LTOT should be followed-up, at least annually, by a clinician experienced in the use of LTOT and the review should include pulse oximetry. Increasingly, these reviews are being undertaken by specialist nurses, who are also able to give patients and their carers valuable psychological and social support.

Patients using concentrators occasionally have problems with drying of the nasal mucosa and soreness from the nasal prongs. A humidifier can be added into the system but great care is needed with its maintenance to prevent infection. Water-based creams such as E45 around the nostrils may reduce soreness. Using nasal prongs can also cause soreness around the ears and across the cheeks, so the oxygen tubing may need to be padded.

Oxygen provision

Changes to oxygen prescribing came into force in February 2006. Prior to this, in England, Wales and Northern Ireland, patients were either prescribed oxygen by their GP without proper assessment or were assessed by the respiratory physician who then had to ask the patient's GP to prescribe a concentrator. This somewhat haphazard system has been replaced with a 'one stop' integrated oxygen service provided by independent oxygen companies contracted to the NHS. These contractors have a 24-hour call-out service to supply, maintain and service all the oxygen equipment. They will also supply the patient with necessary disposables, such as tubing, masks or nasal prongs. There were some well-publicised teething problems with this service when it was first introduced. These have improved but the service continues to have supply and support problems in some areas of the UK.

The major advantage of the changes to oxygen prescribing is that it allows the use of all available oxygen-delivery systems: portable oxygen cylinders, liquid oxygen, conservation devices and ambulatory oxygen systems. Patients can now be assessed and supplied with the system that best suits their needs.

Oxygen is ordered on a Home Oxygen Order Form (HOOF). Whilst GPs are still able to prescribe oxygen, it is anticipated that most prescriptions will be generated from hospitals. The HOOF need be completed only once (unless there is a change to the patient's circumstances) and sent to the contractor. The necessary equipment is then delivered to the patient's home and appropriately maintained and serviced by the contracting company. Oxygen supplies are no longer available on prescription from pharmacies.

The HOOF is completed with the patient and prescriber details. The same form is used to prescribe LTOT, ambulatory and short-burst oxygen therapy. The following information must be provided to the contractor:

- the oxygen flow rate

- the number of hours per day it should be used

- whether nasal prongs or masks are to be used (if masks are requested, the fixed percentage of oxygen delivered through the mask must be stipulated)

- whether humidification is needed

- whether a light-weight cylinder option is required for ambulatory oxygen

- whether a conserving device is contraindicated

- a clinical code indicating the reason for the prescription.

The HOOF is also used to order oxygen supplies for patients going on holiday.

In order for oxygen to be delivered to the patient, their details have to be given to the contractor. Patients will therefore need to sign a consent form, the Home Oxygen Consent Form (HOCF) to allow transfer of data. The signed HOCF is retained and filed with the patient's records.

Cost/benefit

Oxygen is an expensive therapy. In 2002–3 the total cost of oxygen therapy in England and Wales was £34.8 million; £19.8 million for oxygen cylinders and £15.0 million for oxygen concentrators.

There are still far too many patients using oxygen cylinders who may not be gaining any benefit. These patients should all be reviewed and, on the basis of a valid clinical assessment, should either have the oxygen removed- not always easy as patients feel dependent on the oxygen - or the delivery system changed to a concentrator. Undertaking this step should considerably reduce oxygen prescribing costs.

The use of domestic size oxygen cylinders (size F) for 15 hours per day costs around £6,500 per year. The cost of a concentrator is considerably less at £1,500, plus about £80 per month for maintenance and £20 per month for electricity, the cost of which is refunded to the patient. The major expense of the concentrator is the 'one off' installation cost. More appropriate equipment needs to be provided in many cases.

Concentrators are very much more convenient for the patient to use and enable greater mobility around the home. A size F cylinder needs to be changed every 11 hours or so, so spare cylinders must be ordered, delivered and stored. It is not possible to fit long lengths of tubing to a cylinder and the patient is effectively 'chained' to the oxygen source. Any benefits in improved exercise tolerance are therefore likely to be undermined. In contrast, up to 50 metres of tubing can be attached to a concentrator, allowing the patient a considerable degree of mobility around the home.

LTOT prolongs life and has some benefits in health status. A French survey of 13,500 patients using LTOT found that 55% of them were able to wash unaided. However, 25% never left their homes and 25% never went on holiday. The more widespread availability of portable oxygen systems might improve this situation.

Ambulatory oxygen therapy

Ambulatory oxygen is delivered by equipment that can be carried by most patients, thus providing portable oxygen during exercise and daily activity. It is used in two ways:

- As part of LTOT – when the benefits are the same as those of LTOT

- In isolation, during exercise – as a therapy for people who are not chronically hypoxic, in the hope of improving exercise tolerance and quality of life.

The technology for delivering ambulatory oxygen is evolving rapidly. Very lightweight cylinders are now available and oxygen conservation systems can considerably prolong the life of portable cylinders. They are becoming an increasingly practical proposition for extended trips outside the home. Liquid oxygen, however, remains an expensive option and it is still not widely available in all parts of the country.

The Royal College of Physicians Guidelines give the following indications for ambulatory oxygen therapy.

- It can be prescribed for patients on LTOT who are mobile and need to or can leave the home on a regular basis. The type of portable device will depend on the patient's mobility.

- Patients without chronic hypoxaemia and LTOT should be considered for ambulatory oxygen if they show evidence of:
  - exercise oxygen desaturation
  - improvement in exercise capacity and/or dyspnoea with ambulatory oxygen therapy and the motivation to use ambulatory oxygen outside the house.

Assessment for ambulatory oxygen

Ambulatory oxygen should be prescribed only after appropriate assessment by a specialist. The purpose of such assessment is:

- to examine the extent of desaturation and improvement in exercise capacity with supplemental oxygen

- to evaluate the oxygen flow rate that is required to correct exercise desaturation

- to determine the type of ambulatory equipment that best suits the patient's requirements.

Short-burst oxygen

In the past many patients have been prescribed oxygen to be used as required when breathless, or to enable them to perform activities around the house more easily. There have been no clinical studies that show any beneficial role for oxygen used in short-burst format. Some experts are of the opinion that oxygen used in this way is no more than an expensive placebo but, anecdotally, patients often find it beneficial. This may be due to the cooling flow of oxygen on the face and a simple fan may have the same effect.

In essence, short-burst oxygen for COPD is an area of high cost and no real benefit. Patients prescribed oxygen for use in this way might also fit the criteria for LTOT, and consideration should be given to referring them for assessment for this.

The following are the indications from the RCP Guidelines.

- Despite extensive prescription of oxygen for short-burst use, there is no adequate evidence available for firm recommendations.

- Short-burst oxygen should be considered for episodic breathlessness not relieved by other treatments in patients with severe COPD or for palliative care.

- It should be prescribed only if an improvement in breathlessness and/or exercise tolerance can be documented.

The 2010 NICE update recommendations echo those of the Royal College. If short-burst oxygen is required it should be given via oxygen cylinder. If patients use more than three cylinders a month, however, a concentrator may be a more cost-effective option.

Oxygen use in exacerbations in the community and en route to hospital

It has long been recognised that patients who are having exacerbations of COPD may be tipped into respiratory failure and retain carbon dioxide. If such patients are given high concentrations of oxygen in the ambulance on their way to hospital it may suppress respiratory drive and increase mortality. This has led to guidelines being produced which mean that all paramedics now measure oxygen saturations and give titrated oxygen doses to reach a target oxygen saturation of 88–92%. There is now evidence that the use of this procedure reduces mortality.

Patients with known respiratory failure, and particularly with a past history of carbon dioxide retention, are given emergency warning cards by the hospital that will be seen by paramedics to help alert to the need of great care with emergency oxygen.

Non-invasive ventilation (NIV)

NIV is now a well-established and widely available method of providing ventilatory support to patients in respiratory failure due to an exacerbation of COPD. There is now increasing interest in the provision of NIV long term, as a treatment for chronic hypercapnic respiratory failure. In patients already receiving LTOT it has been found to improve:

- daytime $PaCO_2$
- resting dyspnoea (which significantly improved over time)
- quality of life.

It had no significant effect on hospital admissions and, not surprisingly, no effect on lung function.

Several mechanisms have been suggested for the benefit of NIV in stable COPD. It may serve to rest fatigued respiratory muscles allowing recovery of inspiratory muscle function. It may also improve sleep quality by reducing episodes of hypoventilation. By reducing nocturnal hypoventilation it is thought that it may allow the respiratory centre to be 'reset', reducing daytime hypercapnia.

Patients who remain hypercapnic and acidotic on LTOT, or who have required assisted ventilation during an exacerbation may benefit from referral to a specialist centre for consideration of this therapy. It is not widely available, but, with improving technology may become more so in the future.

Travel, flying, and scuba diving

Patients with severe COPD will often require advice about travel, particularly if flying is involved. Aircraft cabin pressures are equivalent to 5000–8000 feet above sea level, which reduces the ambient oxygen pressure to 15–18kPa. In a healthy individual this will reduce mean arterial oxygen from 12kPa to 8.7kPa, with a relatively insignificant drop in oxygen saturation from 96% to 90%. In patients with severe lung disease and hypoxia this reduction in ambient oxygen pressure is likely to cause a potentially hazardous drop in arterial oxygen levels unless they are given supplemental oxygen during the flight.

Other problems may include expansion of emphysematous bullae and abdominal gases resulting in compression of functioning lung. Cabin humidity is reduced on long flights, resulting in potential drying of bronchial secretions.

It has been suggested that, for a patient to be safe to fly:

- the FEV_1 should be in excess of 25% predicted
- the SaO_2 should be greater than 92%
- the pre-flight PaO_2 should be greater than 9.3kPa or 70mmHg
- there should be no hypercapnia.

Airlines often use the yardstick of the person being unable to walk without dyspnoea for more than 50 yards as an indicator of the need for further assessment.

Patients should be encouraged to see a doctor well before they intend to travel so that appropriate tests can be arranged. Airlines need to be approached well in advance and they often require GPs to fill in appropriate data, which a hospital assessment can provide.

The airline will usually ask if a flow rate of 2 or 4 litres per minute should be provided.

Oxygen can be arranged on most scheduled flights by prior arrangement, but the cost can vary from nothing at all to £100 per flight, depending on the airline. It is not available on the budget, 'no frills' airlines.

Patients with recent pneumothorax or emphysematous bullae may also be at increased risk of spontaneous pneumothorax while flying. Travel by land or sea is usually less of a problem.

If there is any doubt about the advisability of air travel, patients should be referred for assessment by a respiratory physician. Some centres can perform a hypoxic challenge by giving patients air with reduced oxygen levels by cylinder in order to assess their response to the reduced oxygen levels they are likely to experience during a flight.

Scuba diving is not recommended for people with COPD.

Surgery

Treatment of emphysematous bullae

A small proportion of COPD patients may develop large cyst-like spaces – bullae – in the lung. These tend to compress the more normal areas of lung, thus reducing their ability to function efficiently. Large bullae can form in relatively normal lung or with any degree of emphysema. It is not clear how bullae originate but it is most likely that an area of local lung degeneration acts as the focus for an enlarging space. Surgery in such cases can significantly improve symptoms and function.

The symptoms produced by bullae are similar to those from the associated underlying emphysema. They can, however, usually be readily detected on a routine chest X-ray. Rarely, they can present as a pneumothorax. Before surgery is considered, there must be careful specialist physiological assessment and anatomical imaging of the bullae and surrounding lung with CT scanning. The best results are usually obtained in younger patients with large bullae and lesser degrees of airflow obstruction. The degree of emphysema in the surrounding lung is an important determinant of the success of this procedure.

There are a number of surgical approaches, ranging from thora-cotomy to a laser technique via a thoracoscope. The aim is to obliterate the abnormal space and restore the elastic integrity of the lung, allowing the compressed areas of the lung to re-expand. Benefits from the surgery are usually felt almost immediately, and the improvement in lung function and symptoms seems to be main-tained. Deterioration after the surgery seems to follow the standard course for a patient with emphysema. Operative mortality is low and should decrease further as the preoperative assessment procedures to screen out unsuitable patients improve.

Surgery to reduce lung volume

Lung volume reduction surgery is a relatively new technique. It was developed in the USA but is gaining in popularity in the UK. The operation is performed through a sternal split and involves one or both lungs. The aim is to remove 20–30% of the most distended emphysematous parts of the lungs. The lungs are then stapled and sutured to prevent air leaks. Complications are not uncommon, particularly relating to air leaks. Operative mortality is, at present, 1–3% depending on the centre. Careful preoperative assessment seems to be the key to success.

Lung volume reduction particularly reduces residual volume, improving vital capacity by 20–40%. FEV_1 can increase by between 20% and 80%, and the six-minute walking distance may improve by 30%. Longer term follow-up shows that the peak effect seems to occur at six to eight months following surgery, after which there is a slow decline. However, after two years most patients will still have better lung function than they had before the surgery.

The large NETT study, performed in the USA, compared outcomes of surgery with medical treatment. Exercise capacity was far superior in the surgical treatment arm, as was lung func-tion, quality of life and dyspnoea. Overall mortality was similar for the two groups although there was a higher initial mortality in the surgical group. The patients who most benefitted were those with upper lobe emphysema and low baseline exercise capability.

A subsequent analysis of the NETT data showed that the surgical group also had a 30% reduction in exacerbation frequency.

This surgical technique is still in its infancy in the UK and many more carefully controlled studies are needed to fully evaluate its usefulness.

An innovative non-invasive technique is currently being developed. It involves the insertion of a one-way valve via a bronchoscope into the airway leading to the worse-affected area of lung. The valve allows air to escape from the lung but will not allow air in. Over a period of a few days the area of lung supplied by that airway collapses, allowing re-expansion of the remaining lung.

Lung transplant

Single lung transplant is the favoured option for emphysema, although double lung transplant procedures can be performed. The operation is generally straightforward and the results are deemed to be excellent. FEV_1 is usually restored to 50% of the predicted value. Lung transplantation is usually offered only to patients under 50 years of age, so the procedure is a likely option for alpha-1 anti-trypsin deficiency emphysema, which presents in this young age group. Generally it is considered only for patients with a life expectancy of less than 18 months. UK survival figures are 60% at three years.

The main drawbacks are related to tissue rejection and immuno-suppressant therapy. A late and serious complication is the development of obliterative bronchiolitis, which occurs in 30% of patients surviving five years. Unfortunately, this widespread inflammatory fibrotic condition of the small airways is frequently fatal at between six and twelve months.

Vaccinations and antiviral drugs

Influenza

Vaccination against influenza is recommended for all elderly patients, and has reduced mortality by 70% in this group. It is also indicated for people with a range of chronic diseases, including COPD, and for anyone with decreased immunity. A Cochrane review in 2008 showed a significant reduction in exacerbations and influenza related respiratory infections. Although there have been few studies in COPD patients as a specific group these positive results, by inference from the data relating to elderly people, demonstrate that there are definite benefits from regular annual vaccination.

Pneumococcus

Streptococcus pneumoniae is the commonest cause of community-acquired pneumonia. Pneumococcal infection is more common in adults over 50 years; in people over 65 years the risk of infection increases by two- to fivefold. The Department of Health includes COPD patients in its at-risk groups for pneumococcal vaccination. Immunisation should be with the polyvalent vaccine, which is a single injection. Immunocompromised or splenectomised patients should be given booster injections every five years.

There are no controlled studies of the effectiveness of this vaccine in COPD, although an evaluation from the USA concluded that the vaccination of people over 65 years is cost saving.

Antiviral drugs

There are currently three antiviral medications available for the treatment and prophylaxis of influenza; amantadine (Lysovir), oseltamivir (Tamiflu) and zanamivir (Relenza). Amantadine is not recommended by NICE, and zanamivir, which is given by inhalation, can cause bronchoconstriction. The drug of choice for COPD patients is the oral therapy, oseltamivir.

Oseltamivir and zanamivir are active against influenza A and B viruses. They are neuraminidase inhibitors that work by preventing the release of virus from infected cells, thus reducing the ability of the virus to replicate and spread. When used to treat influenza they need to be started as soon as possible after the onset of flu-like symptoms, and within 48 hours.

The recommended dose of ostelamivir is 75mg twice daily for 5 days, and for zanamivir 10mg by inhalation twice daily for 5 days. Both drugs have been found to reduce the number of days of symptoms and there is some evidence that they reduce the incidence of complications, such as pneumonia. However, there have been no studies of these therapies in COPD specifically, only in 'at risk' groups, which includes COPD patients.

Oseltamivir and zanamivir can also be used to prevent influenza (post-exposure prophylaxis) for people 'at risk' who have been in contact with someone with influenza and are inadequately protected by vaccination. It must be stressed that the most effective method of preventing influenza is vaccination and it is important to encourage COPD patients to have the vaccine every year. However, antiviral drugs may be used for prophylaxis in influenza outbreaks where the circulating virus is not well matched to the vaccine in use that year, or for those individuals who have not been vaccinated, or in whom the vaccine is contraindicated.

Nutrition

There is some epidemiological evidence suggesting that diets rich in fresh fruit and vegetables are beneficial in slowing the progression of COPD. Such diets are also, of course, valuable in reducing the risk of coronary artery disease and some cancers. It is thought that the high levels of antioxidants in vitamins C and E have a protective effect on lung tissue. However, a study with vitamin E supplements failed to find any significant benefit compared with a placebo. It is also thought that some natural fish oils may protect the lungs through antioxidant enhancement, but scientific evidence for this is lacking.

Obesity

COPD patients who are overweight are likely to have greater impairment of activity and will experience a greater degree of breathlessness than patients of a normal weight. This in turn causes them to lead a more sedentary existence and have a worsened quality of life. You should encourage overweight patients to lose weight as well as to get regular exercise. (See also Chapter 9.)

Malnutrition and muscle wasting

A low body mass index (BMI) and loss of lean muscle mass are common in COPD, especially when emphysema is the predominant pathological problem. It does need to be borne in mind, however, that BMI is a less reliable indicator of nutritional status in older people, than it is in the young. This is due to age-related changes in posture, muscle-to-fat ratio and height. Weight loss, particularly if it is more than 3Kg, needs to be noted and acted on. Weight loss, and a low BMI are poor prognostic signs and increase the risk of death from COPD.

The cause of weight loss in emphysema is complex and poorly understood. It used to be thought that the chronically increased work of breathing, coupled with difficulties in shopping, preparing food and eating when constantly breathless, caused a negative energy balance and, thus, weight loss. This is now thought not to be the sole cause as, in addition to weight loss, most people with COPD have peripheral muscle weakness linked to loss of muscle mass. It has been discovered that there are systemic inflammatory processes and changes in muscle metabolism in these patients.

Raised levels of certain cytokines, including interleukin 8 (IL-8) and tumour necrosis factor alpha (TNF-α), have been found, and these seem likely to have an important role in causing loss of muscle mass. Increased levels of cytokines may be a response to low levels of oxygen in the tissues (tissue hypoxia), resulting from the destruction of alveoli. This might help to explain why weight loss occurs in some patients with comparatively minor FEV_1 impairment and why patients with chronic bronchitis do not seem to have comparable tissue hypoxia and weight loss.

It should be remembered that loss of muscle mass is also a consequence of the muscle deconditioning that occurs from lack of activity.

It is possible – though difficult – to treat and partially reverse this weight loss. Increased exercise, particularly through a programme of pulmonary rehabilitation, coupled with nutritional supplements and, rarely, anabolic steroids have increased both weight and muscle mass. This may result in a small increase in survival rate for patients who gain weight. Non-steroidal anti-inflammatory drugs (NSAIDs) have been used to block the action of the cytokines that may be involved in causing weight loss in patients with terminal cancer, but this does not seem to have been tried in COPD.

Breathlessness can make the very act of eating tiring. Eating can also induce greater breathlessness. Practical advice to patients includes eating small but frequent high-calorie meals. Fish is more digestible than meat and requires less effort to chew. Pureed vegetables and soups also require less effort to consume. Referral to a dietician is recommended by NICE for patients with a low BMI (less than 20) and for those who have lost 3Kg or more. Patients who are prescribed nutritional supplements should also be encouraged to exercise, ideally by referring them for pulmonary rehabilitation.

Exercise

Exercise is an important part of the management of COPD, and is discussed in detail in Chapter 9. Regular exercise is helpful both physically and psychologically, and encourages patients to lead a more normal social life. Encourage patients to regularly walk to the point of breathlessness. Explain that regular walking, pushing themselves a little further each day, will help improve physical fitness. They need reassurance that breathlessness in these circumstances will do no harm to their heart or lungs and is, in fact, positively beneficial. Repeating these positive messages at follow-up visits is helpful.

Psychological and social issues

Depression and anxiety

Many patients with COPD become clinically anxious or depressed, particularly those who have a severe degree of physical impairment or are hypoxic. Those with severe COPD have a 2.5 times greater risk of depression, compared with a healthy population. They may feel embarrassed by their breathlessness or inability to exercise, and therefore may tend not to go out and socialise. They may feel guilty about their inability to perform jobs around the house and garden. Impaired activity levels affect both the patient and their partner, family and carers, and can reduce their ability to socialise, take holidays and enjoy a normal life. Depression, as you would expect, has a detrimental effect on quality of life scores and also leads to an increased risk of hospitalisation.

NICE published guidelines on the management of depression in adults with a chronic physical health problem in 2009. It presents a 'stepped care model' and emphasises that the first step is to identify those patients with depression. There is considerable overlap between the symptoms of depression and COPD. Systematic assessment, as described in Chapter 6, will help ensure that this is not overlooked.

For those with mild-to-moderate depressive symptoms active monitoring and low-intensity psychological and psychosocial interventions, such as a peer support programme, or guided self-help based on the principles of cognitive behavioural therapy (CBT), are appropriate first line interventions. Drug therapy should not be used routinely to treat such individuals, but should be considered if there is a past history of severe depression, or if the mild depression has been present for two or more years. It should also be considered if first line interventions have failed to produce an improvement.

Patients who present with moderate depression, or who have failed to respond to first line therapy should be considered for treatment with standard anxiolytics or antidepressants.

Care should be taken, however, not to prescribe medication that might depress the respiratory drive or interact with existing medication. First choice is a selective serotonin reuptake inhibitor (SSRI), such as citalopram or sertraline. Small amounts of alcohol are acceptable and, for people with severe COPD who have difficulty sleeping, may be preferable to sleeping pills.

Benefits

Patients with more severe symptoms should be advised and encouraged to obtain Social Security benefits, which may help to improve their health status. The Citizens Advice Bureaux and the local Department for Work and Pensions can provide information about entitlement to state benefits and how to apply for them.

- The Blue Badge car parking scheme is probably the most practical benefit. Patients whose exercise capability is less than 100 yards on the flat can qualify for a car badge, which allows parking in many restricted areas – enabling easier access to shops, cinema, theatre, beaches and the countryside.

- There are two main disability benefits: the Disability Living Allowance and Attendance Allowance.

  - Disability Living Allowance covers people who need either personal care or help with getting around, or both, because they are ill or disabled. To qualify, they must have needed help for three months and will need it for at least another six months and also be under 65 years of age when this help was first needed. The award depends on how disabled the Department for Work and Pensions reckons the person is.

  - Attendance Allowance is for people 65 and over who need personal care and have needed that help for at least six months.

- Statutory Sick Pay covers employed people who are sick for more than four days; it can be paid for up to 28 weeks. People who are self-employed or unemployed may, if they have paid enough National Insurance contributions, be entitled to

Incapacity Benefit. The rate depends on the person's age and how long they have been off work.

- People of working age who have not paid enough National Insurance contributions may qualify for Severe Disablement Allowance if they have not been able to work for at least 28 weeks. They must also have been assessed by the Department for Work and Pensions as being 80% disabled in that time.

- Work-related Industrial Injuries Disablement Benefit is for people who have COPD as a result of exposure to, say, coal dust and this has been established as the cause of their disease.

The Breathe Easy Club of the British Lung Foundation charity provides information and support, and has local groups who meet for social and educational benefits. (For contact details, see the entry in the 'Useful addresses' section.)

Severe breathlessness and palliative care

Severe breathlessness

In end-stage COPD, breathlessness may be so severe that eating and talking become difficult and life is distressing for both patient and carer. Bronchodilators in high doses are the first line of therapy, either by large volume spacer or by nebuliser. Oral prednisolone in doses up to 40mg per day may produce initial improvement, but the benefit is usually small. Oxygen in short bursts from a cylinder may be prescribed.

The NICE guidelines have reviewed the evidence for various therapies to help end-stage breathlessness and have made a number of recommendations.

- Opiates can be used for the palliation of breathlessness in end-stage COPD unresponsive to other medical therapy. (A double-blind study supports the use of low-dose sustained-release morphine to improve dyspnoea scores and provide a better quality of sleep.)

- Benzodiazepines, tricyclic antidepressants, major tranquillisers and oxygen should also be used when appropriate.

Palliative care

Palliative care has been defined by the World Health Organization as the active, total care of patients whose disease is not responsive to curative treatment. A palliative approach is multidisciplinary and focused on the control of pain and other symptoms and the provision of psychological, social and spiritual support for the patient, their family and carers.

The management of severe COPD has a large palliative element, yet there is relatively little information about which approaches are most beneficial and, whilst the provision of care is improving, it has been poor and there is much still to be done to raise standards. One study from the UK compared the needs of patients with COPD and of those with lung cancer and found greater problems in the COPD group. The most common symptoms are extreme breathlessness (95%), pain (68%), fatigue (68%), difficulty sleeping (55%) and thirst (55%). Another UK-based qualitative study found that patients experienced a poor quality of life in the last year, that there was little contact with community services (community nurses, social workers), home adaptations were often provided too late to be of benefit and support for bereaved relatives was not always available.

The nature of COPD, slow progression with acute exacerbations, creates problems with the introduction of palliative care. Although the prognosis of patients with severe COPD is poor, there are many individuals for whom the interval from diagnosis to death is measured in years. The slow decline of the disease trajectory (Figure 10.1), compared with the more predictable trajectory of cancer (Figure 10.2) makes accurate prognostication difficult. Deciding on the right moment to discuss 'end of life' issues and palliation with patients and their families can be problematic. Some healthcare professionals feel that such discussions destroy hope, although surveys of patients and their relatives do not support this view. It is a sad fact that there are still occasions when neither the patient nor their relatives are aware of the terminal nature of the patient's condition, appropriate support is not provided, and death comes as a shock.

Palliative care is a difficult area in which to conduct research, but some themes have emerged from the studies that have been done:

- Patients are interested in Advanced Directives, want to have discussions with their doctor about the end of life and want to be fully involved in decision making.

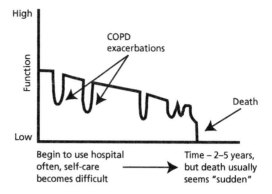

Figure 10.1 Disease trajectory in COPD

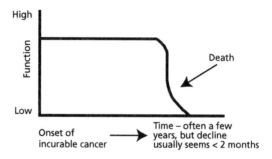

Figure 10.2 Disease trajectory in cancer

- When such discussions have taken place they were most often initiated by the patient.

- The majority of patients want to decide about life-support in the event of hospitalisation. Such discussions are best approached when the patient is stable.

'Knowing' the patient is a vital element in deciding on the best time to raise this sensitive subject, how the conversation should be framed and what is the most appropriate style and content. The nature of general practice, providing patients and their families with continuity of care, probably makes it the best place for these discussions to occur. The use of the Gold Standards Framework to identify patients at the end of life, and its inclusion in the General Medical

Services contract in the UK, has raised the profile of patients with end-stage disease, including those with COPD.

Organisation of palliative care for COPD falls mainly on primary care, with input from hospital respiratory specialists and respiratory nurses, but there has been a far less effective framework than that for cancer services. The need for an effective strategy and structure has been highlighted in the National Clinical Strategy for COPD.

The NICE guideline states that patients with end-stage COPD should have access to the full range of services offered by multidisciplinary palliative care teams, including admission to a hospice.

Further reading

Oxygen therapy

Cooper CB, Waterhouse J, Howard P (1987) Twelve year clinical study of patients with chronic hypoxic cor pulmonale given long-term oxygen therapy. *Thorax* **42**: 105–10

Crockett AJ, Cranston JM, Moss JR, et al. (2001) A review of long-term oxygen therapy for chronic obstructive pulmonary disease. *Respiratory Medicine* **95**(6): 437–43

Dilworth JP, Higgs CMB, Jones PA, et al. (1990) Acceptability of oxygen concentrators; the patients' view. *British Journal of General Practice* **40**: 415–17

Eaton T, Garrett JE, Young P, et al. (2002) Ambulatory oxygen improves quality of life of COPD patients: A randomised controlled study. *European Respiratory Journal* **20**(2): 306–12

Lahdensuo A, Ojanen M, Ahonen A, et al. (1989) Psychological effects of continuous oxygen therapy in hypoxic chronic obstructive pulmonary disease patients. *European Respiratory Journal* **2**: 977–80

Medical Research Council Oxygen Working Party (1981) Report. Long-term domiciliary oxygen therapy in chronic hypoxic cor pulmonale complicating chronic bronchitis and emphysema. *Lancet* **1**: 681–6

Nocturnal Oxygen Therapy Trial Group (1980) Continuous or nocturnal oxygen therapy in hypoxic chronic obstructive lung disease. *Annals of Internal Medicine* **93**: 391–8

Okubadejo AA, Paul EA, Wedzicha JA (1994) Domiciliary oxygen cylinders: indications, prescription and usage. *Respiratory Medicine* **88**(10): 777–85

Roberts CM, Franklin J, O'Neill R, et al. (1998) Screening patients in general practice with COPD for long term domiciliary oxygen requirement using pulse oximetry. *Respiratory Medicine* **92**: 1265–8

Royal College of Physicians of London (1999) *Domiciliary Oxygen Therapy Services. Clinical guidelines and advice for prescribers.* RCP, London

Non-invasive ventilation

Clini E, Sturani C, Rossi A, et al. (2002) The Italian multicentre study on noninvasive ventilation in chronic obstructive pulmonary disease patients. *European Respiratory Journal* **20**(3): 529–38

Meecham Jones DJ, Paul EA, Jones PW, et al. (1995) Nasal pressure support ventilation plus oxygen compared with oxygen therapy alone in hypercapnic COPD. *American Journal of Respiratory & Critical Care Medicine* **152**(2): 538–44

Plant PK, Elliott MW (2003) Management of ventilatory failure in COPD. *Thorax* **58**(6): 537–42

Travel and flying

British Thoracic Society Standards of Care Committee. (2002) Managing passengers with respiratory disease planning air travel. *Thorax* **57**: 289–304

Surgery

Brenner M, McKenna RJ, Gelb AF, et al. (1998) Rate of FEV_1 change following lung reduction surgery. *Chest* **113**: 652–9

McGraw L (1997) Lung volume reduction surgery: an overview. *Heart and Lung* **26**: 131–7

National Emphysema Treatment Trial Research Group (2003) A randomised trial comparing lung-volume-reduction surgery with medical therapy for severe emphysema. *New England Journal of Medicine* **348**: 2059–72

O'Brien GM, Criner GJ (1998) Surgery for severe COPD. Lung volume reduction and lung transplantation. *Postgraduate Medical Journal* **103**: 179–94

Nutrition

National Institute for Clinical Excellence (2006) Nutrition support for adults: oral nutrition support, enteral tube feeding and parenteral nutrition. *Clinical Guideline 32*. Available at www. nice.org.uk/CG32

Schols AMWJ, Slangen J, Volovics L, et al. (1998) Weight loss is a reversible factor in the prognosis of chronic obstructive pulmonary disease. *American Journal of Respiratory and Critical Care Medicine* **157**: 1791–7

Sridhar MK (1995) Why do patients with emphysema lose weight? *Lancet* **345**: 1190–1

Depression and psychosocial issues

National Institute for Health and Clinical Excellence (2009) Depression in adults with a chronic physical health problem. *Clinical Guideline 91*. Available at www.nice.org.uk/CG91

Palliation

Abernethy AP, Currow DC, Firth P, et al. (2003) Randomised, double-blind, controlled crossover trial of sustained-release morphine for the management of refractory dyspnoea. *British Medical Journal* **327**: 523–6

Davis CL (2001) Organising the provision of effective palliative care services for patients with advanced COPD. In Wedzicha PI, Miles A (eds) *The Effective Management of COPD*. Aesculapius Medical Press, London

Department of Health (2005) The Gold Standards Framework. DoH. London. Available at www.goldstandardsframework. Nhs. uk/gp_contract.php

Elkington H, White P, Higgs R, Pettinari CJ (2001) GPs' views of discussions of prognosis in severe COPD. *Family Practitioner* **18**(4): 440-4

Heffner JE, Fahy B, Hilling L, et al. (1996) Attitudes regarding advance directives among patients in pulmonary rehabilitation.

American Journal of Respiratory & Critical Care Medicine **154**(6 Pt 1): 1735–40

Jennings AL, Davies AN, Higgins JPT, et al. (2003) Opioids for the palliation of breathlessness in terminal illness. *The Cochrane Library* **3**(3)

Rhodes P (1999) Focus on palliative care. Palliative care: the situation of people with chronic respiratory disease. *British Journal of Community Nursing* **4**(3): 131–6

Acute exacerbations and referral to hospital

Main points

1 Exacerbations of COPD symptoms are common and tend to occur more frequently with more severe levels of COPD. They usually are more common during the winter months and can last 1–3 weeks, although some exacerbations may take up to three months before patients feel they are back to their baseline. Frequent exacerbations are related to a more rapid decline in lung function and life quality.

2 Exacerbations may be infective, characterised by increasing sputum volume, sputum purulence and breathlessness; or they may be related to changes in airflow obstruction, with increased breathlessness, wheeze and cough.

3 Treatment may include:
   - increased bronchodilators
   - antibiotics
   - a course of oral corticosteroids for one to two weeks.

4 The decision to manage the exacerbation at home or admit the patient to hospital is based on a list of clinical and social factors summarised in Table 11.1.

5 A prolonged worsening of symptoms should raise the suspicion of other diagnoses (e.g. lung cancer) and lead to further investigation such as chest X-ray and possible referral to hospital.

6 There may be other causes of persistent cough, such as chronic nasal catarrh, postnasal drip and bronchiectasis. These should be investigated and treated accordingly.

7 The NICE guidelines support a self-management action plan for COPD with early use of antibiotics and oral steroids.

8 The suspicion of respiratory failure in exacerbations should lead to hospital admission and measurement of arterial blood gases.

9 Criteria for referral to a specialist are listed in Table 11.3.

10 An important part of management of exacerbations is prevention. A range of pharmacological agents are proven to reduce exacerbation frequency, as are pulmonary rehabilitation and vaccinations.

Acute exacerbations of COPD are common and create a large burden on health resources. A UK survey of medical hospital admissions showed that 25% of acute admissions are respiratory, COPD accounting for more than half of these. The average hospital stay is about 7–9 days. Several studies in East London suggest that patients report only 50% of their exacerbations to primary care practitioners.

Exacerbations may also cause a marked worsening of symptoms and quality of life, some patients not recovering to baseline levels for up to three months. More frequent exacerbations may be associated with a more rapid decline in lung function and increased mortality.

Defining an exacerbation

Although exacerbations are common, there is no generally accepted definition of an exacerbation of COPD. An International Consensus Group (Rodriguez-Roisin, 2000) defined an exacerbation as:

> *a sustained worsening of the patient's condition, from the stable state and beyond normal day-to-day variations, that is acute in onset and necessitates a change in regular medication in a patient with underlying COPD.*

Earlier definitions (Anthonisen et al. 1987) have been based on an increase in symptoms of dyspnoea, sputum volume and sputum purulence, with or without symptoms of upper respiratory tract infection.

The NICE guidelines defined an exacerbation as a sustained worsening of the patients' symptoms from their usual stable state, which is rapid in onset. Common symptoms are worsening breathlessness, cough, increased sputum production and change in sputum colour. The change in symptoms often necessitates a change in medication.

Exacerbations become more common with increasing severity of COPD, but can still occur in mild disease. Once patients start to have acute exacerbations, they will continue to have more. Patients who continue to smoke, according to the US Lung Health Study, are more likely to have more exacerbations and also more likely to encourage long-term colonisation of the airways with *Haemophilus influenzae*. Patients with worse health status scores on the St George's Respiratory Questionnaire tend to have more exacerbations and a greater mortality.

The East London study followed a group of 101 patients with moderate to severe COPD for two and a half years and reported a median rate of 2.4 exacerbations per patient per year. Exacerbations occur more commonly during the winter months. Most of them can be managed in the community but more symptomatic patients, or those whose social circumstances are poor, are likely to need admission to hospital.

Common symptoms of exacerbations are:

- increases in sputum purulence (white sputum becoming yellow or green)

- increases in sputum volume

- increased breathlessness, wheeze and chest tightness

- sometimes, fluid retention with ankle swelling

- upper airways symptoms such as colds and sore throats

- reduced exercise tolerance

- fatigue

- acute confusion.

Exacerbations can be triggered in three ways:

1 Infections – both viral and bacterial. According to the East London studies, about 50% of infections are triggered by rhino-viruses and respiratory syncytial viruses, and often start as a cold or upper respiratory infection. However, not all colds lead to exacerbations, and the East London data suggest that only 53% progress to exacerbations. Viral infections tend to cause an exacerbation of longer duration than do bacterial infections.

Symptoms usually include an increase in sputum production and a change in sputum colour to yellow or green, and may be accompanied by a fever. Studies by Stockley's group (2000) in Birmingham examined sputum colour during exacerbations and correlated it with bacterial counts and efficacy of antibiotic treatment. Only deep yellow or green sputum is associated with significant pathological bacterial growth, so antibiotics should be reserved for patients with this pattern of sputum production.

2   Increases in air pollution.

3   A third of exacerbations have no obvious cause but changes occur in lung mechanics and airflow obstruction, such that patients experience greater breathlessness, wheeze and chest tightness but without evidence of infection.

The cause of worsening lung function is frequently not clear. COPD patients often report brief worsening of symptoms on days that are cold, damp or windy but measured lung function on such occasions usually remains unchanged.

Increasing or worsening symptoms may also be caused by other disease processes, and the following should be considered from the history and examination:

- pneumonia

- pneumothorax

- pulmonary oedema

- pulmonary embolism

- lung cancer

- upper airway obstruction or foreign body.

Management of the acute exacerbation

Most exacerbations can be adequately managed in primary care but part of a clinical assessment is to be aware of signs that necessitate admission to hospital. Clinical examination during an acute exacerbation is likely to reveal a patient who is breathless, wheezy and coughing. They may also be cyanosed and have peripheral oedema. A patient who is drowsy, dehydrated or confused is usually in significant respiratory failure and will need urgent admission to hospital. It is helpful to know the patient's usual clinical state so that comparisons can be made. An assessment of the social circumstances and the patient's ability to cope at home are as important as the clinical assessment when making the important decision about whether to manage them at home or to admit them to hospital. Measurement of oxygen saturation with pulse oximetry may be a useful adjunct to assessing exacerbation severity particularly if baseline saturation is known. Generally oxygen saturation below 90% suggests significant hypoxia.

The list below outlines the features of severe exacerbations and Table 11.1 the NICE guidelines' pointers for deciding when a patient needs admission.

The signs and features of severe COPD (NICE update 2010) are:

- marked dyspnoea

- tachypnoea

- purse lip breathing

- use of accessory muscles (sternomastoid and abdominal)

- acute confusion

- new onset cyanosis

- new onset peripheral oedema

- marked reduction in activities of daily living.

Natural history of an exacerbation

The East London cohort studies have provided considerable clinical information on the course and outcomes of exacerbations in moderate and severe COPD. The group of 101 patients were followed for two and a half years with daily symptom diary cards and peak flow readings; 34 of them also recorded daily spirometry. Deterioration in symptoms often occurred without change in peak flow. Falls in lung function were generally small (median fall in peak flow of 6.6 litres/min) and not useful in predicting exacerbations. Larger falls in peak flow were associated with dyspnoea or colds or were related to longer recovery times from the exacerbation.

Table 11.1 Deciding whether to treat an acute exacerbation at home or in hospital

Criteria	Treat at home	Treat in hospital
Able to cope at home	Yes	No
Breathlessness	Mild	Severe
General condition	Good	Poor, deteriorating
Level of activity	Good	Poor, confined to bed
Cyanosis	No	Yes
Worsening peripheral oedema	No	Yes
Level of consciousness	Normal	Impaired
Already receiving LTOT	No	Yes
Social circumstances	Good	Living alone/not coping
Acute confusion	No	Yes
Rapid rate of onset	No	Yes
Significant co-morbidity (particularly cardiac and insulin-dependent diabetes)	No	Yes
Oxygen saturation below 90%	No	Yes
Also available at hospital		
Changes on the chest X-ray	No	Present
Arterial pH level	>7.35	<7.35
Arterial Pao$_2$	>7kPa	<7kPa
Local availability of hospital-at-home services	Yes	No

The more referral indicators that are present, the more likely the need for admission to hospital.

The median time to recovery of peak flow was six days, and of symptoms seven days. However, at 35 days peak flow had returned to normal in only 75%; at 91 days, 7% had still not returned to their baseline lung function. Prolonged recovery was linked to increased dyspnoea and colds.

In patients with frequent exacerbations there are higher basal levels of inflammatory markers, such as interleukins IL-6 and 8, in the lung. As the severity of COPD increases, there seem to be greater levels of persistent bacterial colonisation of the airways and, accordingly, more inflammatory markers. Each of these is associated with more rapid decline in FEV_1. A recently published longitudinal study from the East London group has shown that, over time, patients experiencing frequent exacerbations have more symptoms of longer duration and have a longer recovery time to baseline.

The effect of exacerbations on quality of life was also assessed. Patients with more frequent exacerbations (more than three per year) had significantly worse quality of life than those with fewer exacerbations. This suggests that exacerbation frequency is an important determinant of health status in COPD and, therefore, an important outcome measure.

The original study of Fletcher and Peto in the 1970s suggested that exacerbations made little difference to the rate of decline in FEV_1 over long periods of time. The East London studies and also the Copenhagen City study challenge this conclusion and infer that exacerbations may accelerate the decline in FEV_1.

Patients admitted to hospital with exacerbations have a high readmission rate of 34%, and mortality of 14% at 3 months. While the length of stay in hospital is falling, overall hospital admissions are not. Once exacerbations start the risk of death is 21% at 1 year and 55% at 5 years.

Treatment in the community

Antibiotics

It is common practice to prescribe antibiotics for infective exacerbations of COPD. A meta-analysis of the use of antibiotics compared with a placebo revealed a small but statistically significant benefit in the group treated with antibiotics. The greatest benefit is seen in those with more severe COPD.

The criteria for using antibiotics should include one or more of the following:

- purulent sputum (the most important criterion)
- increased sputum volume.

The most common pathogen is *Haemophilus influenzae*, with *Streptococcus pneumoniae* and *Moraxella catarrhalis* found less commonly. Occasionally, *Chlamydia pneumoniae* is found. The most appropriate antibiotic should follow local microbiology guidelines but standard antibiotics such as amoxycillin, erythromycin and tetracycline, all for seven days, are normally satisfactory. Sputum culture is not usually indicated.

Bronchodilators

For both infective and non-infective exacerbations, the dose of beta-2 agonist and/or anticholinergic inhaled bronchodilators should be increased, or started four-hourly if the patient is not already taking a bronchodilator. Multiple doses of inhaled bronchodilators are safe and can be administered to very breathless patients via a spacer. It is rare that a nebuliser is needed for acute attacks, as high doses of bronchodilator via a spacer have been shown to be just as effective.

Oral corticosteroids

Oral corticosteroids were of significant benefit in exacerbations in two randomised placebo-controlled trials. Both studies showed a more rapid improvement in lung function and symptoms and a shorter hospital stay in the group treated with corticosteroids. Treatment failures were fewer and the time to the next exacerbation was extended in the steroid group.

Corticosteroids may be helpful in exacerbations not caused by infection, where lung function has deteriorated significantly. Oral corticosteroids are of benefit in patients who have increased breathlessness that interferes with their ability to undertake normal activities of daily living. They may also be added to antibiotics for an infection accompanied by marked wheeze and breathlessness. A course of prednisolone 30mg per day is given for 7–14 days and is usually then discontinued unless the patient has failed to recover fully.

Patients already on long-term oral corticosteroids should have the dose increased to 30–40mg per day; on recovery the dose should be reduced over several weeks back to the previous baseline level.

Mucolytics

The new agent erdosteine is licensed only for use in exacerbations in patients with chronic bronchitis. Its role is related to helping patients with thick sputum that is difficult to expectorate. A course of treatment is for 10 days.

Follow-up

Exacerbations treated in the community normally respond well to the therapy outlined above. Patients who fail to respond need further examination and review. An important differential diagnosis to exclude in a patient who is slow in responding is lung cancer. If this is suspected, a chest X-ray should be performed and consideration given to referral to a respiratory specialist.

Follow-up is a good opportunity to assess the patient's clinical state, treatment, inhaler technique, adherence to therapy and psychosocial status. It is also an opportunity for patient education, discussing a self–management plan and messages about smoking, weight loss and exercise.

Recurrent exacerbations

Someone with severe COPD may have many exacerbations in a year. The presence of persistent purulent sputum, perhaps with inspiratory coarse crackles – particularly at the lung bases – may suggest a diagnosis of bronchiectasis.

A study by O'Brien et al. (2002) in Birmingham examined the physiological and radiological (high-resolution CT scan) features of 110 patients presenting to their GP with an acute exacerbation of COPD. There was CT scan evidence of bronchiectasis in 29%, and in 51% radiological emphysema. Only 5% had reversibility levels to suggest asthma. The entry criteria for the study involved sputum production; it is likely that, in a more random selection of COPD patients where irreversible airflow is the main criterion, the prevalence of bronchiectasis would be lower. However, the study serves to underline the heterogeneous nature of COPD and the need to be alert to the possibility of coexisting bronchiectasis. Alternatively, and fairly rarely, patients may have an immune deficiency syndrome or abnormality of cilial function (immotile cilia syndrome).

Persistent nasal catarrh and postnasal drip can cause a productive cough. Treating the nose with decongestants and/or a course of betamethasone and neomycin nose drops, given with the correct technique, may clear the nose and reduce the cough.

Prevention of acute exacerbations

We have seen that exacerbations severely impair quality of life, may speed the rate of decline in lung function, are a major cause of GP consultations and hospital admissions and also are the greatest healthcare burden on the community. Preventing or reducing the severity or duration of an exacerbation is therefore an important goal in the management of COPD.

Many of the therapies in current use will reduce the frequency of exacerbations (see Table 11.2). Self-management action plans, by early intervention with self-held medication, and patient education are a standard part of therapy both to reduce the severity and duration of an exacerbation.

- Vaccination against influenza is of proven benefit both in reducing deaths and respiratory illnesses such as flu and pneumonia. Pneumococcal vaccination has been studied in a group of elderly people with chronic chest disease and was seen to reduce hospitalisations for influenza and pneumonia by 43% and all cause mortality by 29%. Both are recommended by NICE and the Chief Medical Officer.

- Inhaled corticosteroids reduce the number and rate of exacerbations but only in more moderate to severe COPD. The dose-response effect of this action has not yet been studied.

- All LABAs, including the new indacterol, have reduced exacerbation frequency by 12–20%. Similar benefit is seen with tiotropium.

- Combined LABA/inhaled corticosteroid combinations have an additive effect with reduced frequency of over 30% in some studies.

- The new PDE4 inhibitor, rifluomast and theophyllines have some smaller benefits than combined drugs.

- Mucolytics such as carbocisteine and mecysteine reduce exacerbation frequency by 21% according to the latest Cochrane meta-analysis.

- Pulmonary rehabilitation, as well as improving quality of life, results in fewer hospital admissions and less frequent exacerbations.

Table 11.2 Summary of treatment benefits for reducing exacerbation frequency

Intervention	Reduces exacerbations/ hospital admissions*	Improve quality of life/functional capacity
Pulmonary rehabilitation	YES	YES
Long-acting bronchodilator	YES	YES
Long-acting beta agonist/inhaled corticosteroid (in those with FEV_1 <50% and exacerbations	YES	YES

*All by about 25%

Long-term antibiotics

There have been a number of recent studies looking at the effect of longer term antibiotics on reduced exacerbation frequency. One, by Seemungal et al. (2008), gave erythromycin 250mg twice daily over 12 months to 109 patients. There was a 35% reduction in exacerbations in the treatment arm and exacerbations were significantly shorter and probably less severe. Macrolide antibiotics are known to have anti-inflammatory properties which may have contributed to the beneficial result. Previous studies show conflicting results and NICE, in the 2010 update, state that this form of therapy can not at present be recommended. There are more studies in progress which should shed more light on this area.

Self-management

Self-management plans for people with asthma have improved symptoms, reduced exacerbations, achieved higher levels of health status and reduced time off school or work. Patients are given more control of their disease and are instructed to respond early to changes in symptoms. A combination of monitoring of symptoms and of peak flow allows patients to act on any deterioration of asthma rapidly and effectively.

In COPD, as in asthma, the key component of a self-management plan is thorough personalised education about the disease process and the symptoms and changes to be aware of when an exacerbation is occurring. A self-management card should be completed with the patient for them to take away and keep in a readily accessible place at home. A supply of appropriate antibiotics and prednisolone should be prescribed for emergency use. There is good evidence that early intervention with patient-held therapy when an exacerbation is starting will reduce the severity and duration of the attack and may prevent a hospital admission.

An analysis of the effectiveness of self-management plans have been examined by two Cochrane reviews. The first on *Self-Management Education*, published in 2008, examined 14 trials but often with very heterogeneous background designs. There was a significant reduction in hospital admissions by 36% relative to usual care – a NNT of 10 for patients with a higher risk of exacerbation. There were also improvements in quality-of-life scores and a mild reduction in dyspnoea. There were no effects on emergency room visits, days lost from work or lung function.

The second review based on *Action Plans* published in 2005 concluded that plans aid patients in recognising and reacting appropriately to an exacerbation but there were no significant changes of healthcare utilisation.

Some studies, particularly that of Bourbeau et al. (2003), show much more positive results but this study did include a form of pulmonary rehabilitation as part of the intervention arm. Hospital admissions were reduced by 40%, with a 41% reduction in emergency room visits, and there were significant improvements in the impact scale of the St George's Respiratory Questionnaire. Symptoms did not differ between intervention and control groups.

A new large study from the USA (Rice et a.l 2010) of 743 patients with severe COPD compared usual treatment with education, an action plan and monthly follow up. After one year COPD related hospitalisations and emergency room visits were 0.82 per patient in usual care and only 0.48 per patient in intervention (p<0.001). Analysed separately hospital admissions were less but just failed to reach statistical significance. Admissions for other than COPD causes were reduced by 49% and emergency room visits were reduced by 27%. The intervention group had a slower decline in quality of life by more than the clinically important 4 points over one year compared with usual treatment.

NICE and other Guidelines recommend the widespread use of action plans particularly in patients who are having regular exacerbations.

NICE recommendations on self-management

Patients at risk of exacerbations should be given self-management advice in terms of an action plan that encourages them to respond promptly to the symptoms of an exacerbation.

- Start oral steroids if breathlessness increases and interferes with activities of daily living.

- Start antibiotics if sputum becomes purulent.

- Adjust bronchodilator therapy to control symptoms.

Suitable patients should be prescribed a supply of antibiotics and prednisolone to keep at home for use as part of the self-management strategy. They should be advised to contact a healthcare professional if they do not improve.

Stockley et al. have developed a credit-card-sized sputum colour chart for patients to help them to tell when a significant infection is present – i.e. when the sputum is green. There are now many local variations on self-management action plans, one of which, used in Plymouth, is shown in Figure 11.1. A comprehensive self-care booklet has been produced by the British Lung Foundation.

Met Office and anticipatory care plans

COPD patients will tell you that the weather affects them and there is evidence that this is indeed the case. Temperature, humidity and season are the main drivers for the variation in COPD symptoms and severity during the year. Cold temperatures have a direct effect – there is a significant rise in COPD admissions 10–14 days after a fall in temperature below 4⁰C for at least 3 days. Atmospheric 'mixing' affects viral concentrations – higher levels of atmospheric 'mixing' are associated with cyclonic weather conditions and can reduce the winter virus load.

The Met Office has developed a model, collating weather patterns, hospital admission, air quality and infectious disease data, which is used to predict periods when the risk of COPD exacerbations is high. Several other parameters can be added to the model so that it is specific to a particular area.

WHAT ACTION TO TAKE IF YOUR SYMPTOMS GET WORSE:

Step 1

Check the colour of your sputum:

Cough sputum onto a white tissue.

If your sputum colour has changed from clear or pale to a darker shade e.g. yellow or green : **start ANTIBIOTICS.**

RELIEVER TREATMENT

via Inhaler or Nebuliser

Maximum dose........ /........ times per day

Maximum dose........ /........ times per day

ANTIBIOTICS

Please take your home supply **or** obtain a prescription without delay from the surgery.

PREDNISOLONE

Take 30mg once daily (6 x 5mg tablets) For 5–10 days.

Step 2   Look at table

Symptoms	OK	CAUTION	ACTION
Breathless-ness	Normal/ Usual	Worse than usual	Much worse than usual
Cough	Normal/ Usual	More than usual	Much more than usual

If all of your symptoms are in the green OK column continue usual treatment.

If any of your symptoms are in the orange CAUTION column:
Increase your **RELIEVER TREATMENT**, take regular up to maximum dose. Keep a close eye on your symptoms, if you improve within 2 days resume usual treatment.

If NO improvement start PREDNISOLONE.

If any of your symptoms are in the red **ACTION** column

Take maximum reliever treatment **and** start **PREDNISOLONE immediately.**

WARNING

At any time if you get

Severe symptoms:
If you have symptoms in the red ACTION column, have tried medication and you are not getting better, please **contact your doctor/nurse for an urgent appointment.**

EMERGENCY

If you have any of the following:
- Very short of breath
- Chest pains
- High fever
- Feeling of agitation, fear, drowsiness or confusion

DIAL 999 AMBULANCE

Oxygen

In an emergency please do not use **high flow oxygen.**
Give sufficient oxygen to reach the target saturation: .... - ......%
(usual range 88–92%)

Figure 11.1 The Plymouth action plan. Reproduced with permission from Dr Rupert Jones

The Met Office COPD Health Forecasting Service has two main components, the health forecast and anticipatory care. In areas that subscribe to the service COPD patients are given a pack at the beginning of winter, containing lots of guidance on self-care and an action plan. The forecast is sent weekly (and updated during the week). When the forecast indicates a high risk of exacerbation, patients can be contacted and their self-management advice reinforced. A variety of different methods for contacting patients, depending on the area and resources available, have been used:

- Local media (newspapers, local radio)

- Posters in pharmacies, post offices, etc

- SMS text messages

- Automated telephone calls

- Calls from the GP surgery.

Data to be published shortly suggests that this service has had a significant effect in reducing hospital admissions.

Other systems of anticipatory care are being set up with community specialist nurse teams who regularly visit higher risk patients, follow up hospital admissions and supervise patient education and oxygen services. The use of telemedicine is being explored.

Hospital-at-home schemes for acute exacerbations

There is a growing trend for patients with acute exacerbations of COPD who are admitted to hospital to have an initial assessment and, if they are suitable, to be returned home and managed by regular visits from a respiratory nurse team from the hospital.

Patients are examined and undergo investigations such as chest x-ray, oxygen saturation, blood gases and spirometry; enquiries are also made about their social circumstances and mental state. Those who are felt to be affected less severely and are socially suitable are returned home and managed by a respiratory nurse who visits daily until their recovery or will readmit them to hospital if their condition deteriorates. Alternatively, some patients who are admitted to hospital may be suitable for early discharge and nurse-supervised home management.

Controlled studies of hospital-at-home schemes have shown that outcomes such as clinical complications and readmission rates are comparable to those treated in hospital. Patients seem to be very satisfied with being treated at home by a nurse.

Respiratory failure

Respiratory failure is a clinical state characterised by severe hypoxia (PaO_2 less than 7.3kPa), with or without accompanying hypercapnia. The diagnosis is made by measurement of arterial blood gases.

Respiratory failure may accompany exacerbations of COPD. Clinical suspicion of hypoxia includes cyanosis and breathlessness. A raised level of arterial carbon dioxide causes symptoms of central nervous system depression with drowsiness, coma, confusion and mood change. There may also be symptoms of tremor and flap of the hands, muscle jerks and convulsions. The vasodilator effect of raised carbon dioxide results in a bounding pulse, flushed skin and headache, sometimes related to papilloedema. Such patients will always need urgent admission to hospital.

Great care must be taken with oxygen therapy on the way to hospital. Too high a level of inspired oxygen can remove hypoxic respiratory drive and lead to respiratory arrest. The guidelines for the use of oxygen in this situation are described in Chapter 10. On a practical level, if there is no access to pulse oximetry, inspired oxygen of 28% via Venturi mask or 2 litres per minute via nasal cannulae is the maximum that is safe to use at home while waiting for an ambulance.

Treatment of associated conditions

Patients with severe COPD frequently develop pulmonary hypertension and cor pulmonale, usually presenting as peripheral oedema. The addition of diuretics and possibly an ACE inhibitor is indicated in patients with:

- peripheral oedema
- a raised jugular venous pressure
- gallop heart rhythm.

There is no effective therapy for pulmonary hypertension alone but patients with cor pulmonale and right heart failure may benefit from long-term oxygen therapy (LTOT).

Consideration of specialist referral

The indications for specialist referral include:

- to make a diagnosis
- to perform spirometry
- to exclude other possible diagnoses such as lung cancer
- to assess for oxygen therapy or long-term nebuliser treatment
- to offer special advice to younger patients with alpha-1 anti-trypsin deficiency.

The indications for specialist referral as set out in the NICE guidelines are listed in Table 11.3

Table 11.3 Indications for specialist referral

Reason	*Purpose*
Therapeutic advice	
Suspected severe COPD	Confirm diagnosis and optimise therapy
Onset of cor pulmonale	Confirm diagnosis and optimise therapy
Assessment for oxygen therapy	Optimise therapy and measure blood gases
Assessment for nebuliser therapy	Exclude inappropriate prescriptions
Assessment for oral corticosteroids	Justify need for long-term treatment or to supervise withdrawal
Bullous lung disease	Identify candidates for surgery
A rapid decline in FEV_1	Encourage early intervention
Diagnostic advice	
Aged under 40 years or a family history of alpha-1 antitrypsin deficiency	Identify alpha-1 antitrypsin deficiency; consider therapy and screen family
Uncertain diagnosis	Make a diagnosis
Symptoms disproportionate to lung function deficit	Look for other explanations
Frequent infections	Exclude bronchiectasis

Further reading

Anthonisen NR, Manfreda J, Warren CPW, et al. (1987) Antibiotic therapy in exacerbations of chronic obstructive pulmonary disease. *Annals of Internal Medicine* **106**: 196–204

Bourbeau J, Julien M, Maltais F, et al. (2003) Reduction of hospital utilization in patients with chronic obstructive pulmonary disease – A disease specific self management intervention. *Archives of Internal Medicine* **163**: 585–91

Burge S, Wedzicha JA (2003) COPD exacerbations: definitions and classifications. *European Respiratory Journal* **21** (suppl 21): 46s–53s

Davies L, Angus RM, Calverley PMA (1999) Oral corticosteroid in patients admitted to hospital with exacerbations of COPD: a prospective randomised trial. *Lancet* **354**: 456–60

Donaldson GC, Seemugal TAR, Patel IS, et al. (2003) Longitudinal changes in the nature, severity and frequency of COPD exacerbations. *European Respiratory Journal* **22**: 931–6

Effing TW, Monninkhof EM, van der Valk P, et al. (2008) Self management education for patients with chronic obstructive pulmonary disease. *Cochrane Database of Systemic Reviews 2007* **3**

Monninkhof EM, van der Valk P, van der Palen J, et al. (2003) Self-management education for patients with chronic obstructive pulmonary disease: a systematic review. *Thorax* **58**: 394–8

Niewoehner DE, Erbland ML, Deupree RH, et al. (1999) Effect of systemic glucocorticoids on exacerbations of COPD. *New England Medical Journal* **340**: 1941–7

O'Brien C, Guest PJ, Hill SL, Stockley RA (2000) Physiological and radiological characteristics of patients diagnosed with chronic obstructive pulmonary disease in primary care. *Thorax* **55**: 635–42

Rice KL, Dewan N, Bloomfield HA, et al. (2010) Disease management program for chronic obstructive pulmonary disease: a randomised controlled trial. *American Journal of Respiratory and Critical Care Medicine* **182**: 890–6

Rodriguez-Roisin R (2000) Towards a consensus definition for COPD exacerbations. *Chest* **117**: 398S–401S

Saint S, Bent S, Grady D (1995) Antibiotics in COPD: a meta-analysis. *Journal of the American Medical Association* **273**: 957–60

Seemungal TAR, Donaldson GC, Paul EA, et al. (1998) Effect of exacerbation on quality of life in patients with COPD. *American Journal of Respiratory and Critical Care Medicine* **157**: 1418–22

Seemungal TAR, Donaldson GC, Bhowmik A, et al. (2000) Time course and recovery of exacerbations in patients with COPD. *American Journal of Respiratory and Critical Care Medicine* **161**: 1608–13

Seemungal TA, Wilkinson TM, Hurst JR, et al. (2008) Long-term erythromycin therapy is associated with decreased chronic obstructive pulmonary disease exacerbations. *American Journal of Respiratory and Critical Care Medicine* **178**: 1139–47

Stockley RA, O'Brien C, Pye A, Hill SL (2000) Relationship of sputum colour to nature and outpatient management of acute exacerbations of COPD. *Chest* **117**: 1638–45

Turnock AC, Walters EH, Walters JAE, et al. (2005) Action plans for chronic obstructive pulmonary disease. *Cochrane Database of Systemic Reviews 2005* **4**

The 2010 NICE update, GOLD 2009, The National Clinical Strategy and NICE Quality Standards

THE NICE GUIDELINE UPDATE 2010

The National Clinical Guideline Centre for acute and chronic diseases at the Royal College of Physicians have, on behalf of NICE, updated their Guideline on COPD, first published in 2004. There have been changes in diagnosis, spirometric criteria, new airflow obstruction severity levels, an expanded checklist for assessing clinical disease severity and changes in management, which reflect both new innovations and the need for concordance with other major world guidelines.

The new Guideline emphasises the clinical features of COPD rather than an over-reliance on spirometry. Many new recommendations are made based on the persistence of symptoms, including exacerbations, and not on arbitrary levels of lung function.

Treatment and care should be centred on the patient, taking into account their individual needs and preferences. More time is needed to educate the patient about their illness and to provide information on what to do if an exacerbation occurs. Later in the illness patients and carers need to be involved in discussions about outcomes and the options of care available.

Multidisciplinary teams, which should include specialist respiratory nurses, are recommended for best COPD care.

Diagnosis

The update has expanded the criteria around considering a diagnosis of COPD. A diagnosis remains a combination of persistent symptoms in persons over 35 who, in the UK, are smokers or ex-smokers, together with confirmation of airflow obstruction with spirometry.

The symptoms suggestive of COPD in those over 35 years are:

- exertional breathlessness
- chronic cough
- regular sputum production
- frequent winter bronchitis
- wheeze
- without clinical features of asthma:
  - chronic unproductive cough
  - significantly variable breathlessness
  - night-time waking with breathlessness or wheeze
  - significant diurnal or day to day variability of symptoms.

Where COPD is suspected there is also a need to ask about the following:

- weight loss
- effort intolerance
- waking at night
- ankle swelling
- fatigue
- occupational hazards – particularly exposure to dusts
- chest pain
- haemoptysis
- previous TB, particularly in people coming from Asia.

In those suspected of having COPD, spirometry should be performed. The new recommendation is that this should be **post–bronchodilator.** This is in accord with the latest QOF criteria. The absolute and percent predicted vales of FEV_1 and FVC, and the FEV_1/FVC ratio should be recorded. From these values an assessment of COPD severity can be made.

Another new recommendation is to **consider alternative diagnoses** in:

- Older people without typical symptoms of COPD and a FEV_1/ FVC ratio <0.7

- Younger people with symptoms of COPD and a FEV_1 / FVC ratio >0.7

Reversibility testing is not usually necessary as part of the diagnostic process or to plan therapy. However in reality, you would normally perform spirometry as an initial screening tool and, if this is abnormal, will go on to give a bronchodilator to give a definitive, post-bronchodilator spirometric reading – in effect, a reversibility test.

Other tests recommended by NICE on initial diagnosis include:

- a chest X-ray to exclude other diagnoses, particularly lung cancer. Any abnormalities are often best investigated by CT scan and are likely to need referral

- full blood count to look for anaemia and polycythaemia

- BMI.

If the diagnosis is confirmed, appropriate treatment should be started. If the diagnosis is still in doubt, particularly if asthma is suspected, the patient will need to be reassessed after a period of treatment. In essence:

- Clinically significant COPD is **not** present if the FEV_1 and FEV_1/FVC ratio return to normal with drug therapy
- Asthma may be present if :
  - There is a greater than 400ml increase in FEV_1 with bronchodilators
  - Serial PEFs show a significant (more than 20%) diurnal or day-to-day variability
  - There is a greater than 400ml increase in FEV_1 with prednisolone 30mg/day for 2 weeks.

Further tests and investigations may be needed in such cases.

Spirometry

Spirometry remains the gold standard for measuring airflow obstruction and, as such, for confirming the diagnosis of COPD.
Screening is discussed in more depth in the National Strategy but some practices in the UK are performing spirometry on high-risk groups, such as smokers, even if they are asymptomatic. Screening of patients with a symptom such as cough will give a high yield of positive results.

- Spirometry should be performed in people with chronic bronchitis.

- All health professionals involved in the care of people with COPD should have access to spirometry and be able to interpret the results.

- Any health worker with up-to-date training can perform spirometry.

- Spirometry services should have quality control processes.

- Health professionals need to be aware that the use of ERS 1993 reference values (used by all commercial spirometers) may lead to over-diagnosis in older people and are not applicable in black and Asian populations.

Determining disease severity

Spirometry is the definitive way of diagnosing airflow obstruction and the FEV_1% predicted gives a measure of disease severity. Spirometric indices do not, however, correlate well with disability in COPD. NICE has thus produced **a new list of other factors** that should be assessed, as necessary, to provide a more complete picture of the patient's symptoms and quality of life.

- severity of airflow obstruction – FEV_1

- breathlessness – MRC dyspnoea scale

- gas transfer factor – TLco – measured in hospital lung function labs

- health status – perhaps most conveniently assessed in primary care with the new CAT score (see Chapter 6)

- frequency of exacerbations

- exercise capability

- BMI score

- oxygen saturation – pulse oximetry

- presence of symptoms of cor pulmonale.

In some patients the degree of breathlessness seems much greater than would be anticipated from their FEV_1. This needs further investigation, including gas transfer factor, which measures alveolar function, or CT scan. Patients with predominant emphysema may, in the earlier phase of their disease, have widespread alveolar damage with fewer changes in the airways. This could manifest as mild airflow obstruction but with significantly reduced gas transfer and perhaps reduced oxygen saturation. Such change may also be visible on CT scan.

The 2010 NICE update now suggests stages of severity that are in line with the GOLD Guidelines (see Table 6.2). There are a number of riders and important considerations with this new, GOLD-style severity table.

1   Using an FEV_1/FVC ratio below 0.7 as the main determinant of airflow obstruction tends to overestimate the number of diagnosed patients, particularly in the older age groups, when compared with other calculations which are deemed more accurate, such as Lower Limit of Normal (LLN) 5%. For this reason NICE stipulates that for **Stage 1, only those patients with symptoms should be diagnosed with COPD.** The evidence suggests that patients at Stage 1 who are asymptomatic behave like normal individuals and do not show a more rapid decline in FEV_1. NICE discuss in some detail the potential of changing to the below 5% LLN reference values as the main determinant of airflow obstruction. These remove the problem over-diagnosis of elderly patients, but at present there are insufficient data available. This change is likely to occur in the future.

2   Stage 4 very severe should also include patients with respiratory failure who have a FEV_1 below 50%.

3   In the section on the management of stable disease, the choice of therapies is far less based on an arbitrary cut-off of $FEV_1\%$ predicted of 50%, and is more based on the degree of symptoms.

Management of stable disease

There have been a number of important pharmacological and clinical studies since the last Guideline and the Update makes the following recommendations on treatment.

1 Offer once daily LAMA (tiotropium) in preference to four times daily SAMA to patients who remain breathless despite using short-acting bronchodilators as required.

2 In patients with stable COPD who remain breathless, or who have exacerbations despite short-acting bronchodilators as required, offer the following maintenance therapy;

- If FEV_1 greater than 50% predicted , either a LABA or LAMA
- If FEV_1 less than 50% predicted, either LABA and inhaled corticosteroid (ICS) in combination, or LAMA.

3 In patients with FEV_1 greater than 50% predicted who remain breathless or have exacerbations despite maintenance with a LABA

- Consider LABA +ICS combination inhaler
- Consider LAMA in addition to LABA where ICS is declined or not tolerated

4 Offer LAMA in addition to LABA + ICS to those who remain breathless or have exacerbations despite taking LABA+ICS, irrespective of their FEV_1.

5 Consider LABA+ICS in combination in addition to LAMA for patients who remain breathless or have exacerbations despite maintenance therapy with LAMA, irrespective of their FEV_1.

6 Be aware that patients who are taking regular high dose ICS are more at risk of developing pneumonia.

See also Table 8.1 in the pharmacotherapy chapter (Chapter 8).

These recommendations recognise the need for symptomatic treatment at any level of FEV_1% predicted, and the need to step up therapy at an earlier stage. There is evidence that earlier treatment with long-acting bronchodilators and ICS can reduce exacerbations and perhaps prolong life when given at the milder stages of COPD.

There was also a review of mucolytic agents with the recommendation that they should not be routinely used for the purpose of reducing frequency of exacerbations.

The new drug, varenicline has been added to the therapies to aid smoking cessation.

Pulmonary rehabilitation

NICE confirm that pulmonary rehabilitation should be offered to all those patients who consider themselves functionally disabled by COPD – usually MRC dyspnoea grade 3 or above. The new recommendation is that pulmonary rehabilitation should be made available to all appropriate patients with COPD, including those with a recent hospital admission for an acute exacerbation.

Self-management advice

The Update has reviewed new data on self-management schemes and, although more trials are needed to provide a more complete picture, a Grade A evidence level has still been given to the following recommendation. Patients at risk of having an exacerbation of COPD should be given self–management advice that encourages them to respond promptly to the symptoms of an exacerbation. This would normally include having emergency supplies of oral corticosteroids and an antibiotic at home. Patients should have a written management plan to provide guidance on what steps to take when symptoms of an exacerbation occur.

Exacerbations

A detailed review of exacerbation management was not undertaken in this Update and most of the recommendations are unchanged from the 2004 Guideline. The table for deciding if a patient needs admission to hospital or not has been slightly modified (Table 12.1).

Table 12.1 Decision on where to treat patients during an exacerbation

Factor	Treat at home	Treat in hospital
Able to cope at home	Yes	No
Breathlessness	Mild	Severe
General condition	Good	Poor/deteriorating
Level of activity	Good	Poor/confined to bed
Cyanosis	No	Yes
Worsening peripheral oedema	No	Yes
Level of consciousness	Normal	Impaired
Already receiving LTOT	No	Yes
Social circumstances	Good	Living alone/not coping
Acute confusion	No	Yes
Rapid rate of onset	No	Yes
Significant co-morbidity (particularly cardiac and insulin-dependent diabetes)	No	Yes
$SaO_2 <90\%$	No	Yes
Changes on chest radiograph	No	Present
Arterial pH level	7.35	<7.35
Arterial PaO_2	7 kPa	<7 kPa

Referral to a specialist

The table of reasons for referral to a specialist has been updated (Table 12.2).

Follow up in primary care

An important part of the good management of COPD in Primary care is regular, systematic follow up and patient review. This could often be performed in the autumn and could be combined with influenza vaccination, making sure the patient has a self-management plan and has advice about how best to cope with winter conditions, when most exacerbations are likely to occur. Review should, ideally, also include an enquiry about quality of daily living – such as the CAT score – and questions on psychological state, to identify anxiety and depression. Table 12.3 summarises the NICE guidance.

Table 12.2 The updated reasons for referral to a specialist

Reason	Purpose
There is diagnostic uncertainty	Confirm diagnosis and optimise therapy
Suspected severe COPD	Confirm diagnosis and optimise therapy
The patient requests a second opinion	Confirm diagnosis and optimise therapy
Onset of cor pulmonale	Confirm diagnosis and optimise therapy
Assessment for oxygen therapy	Optimise therapy and measure blood gases
Assessment for long-term nebuliser therapy	Optimise therapy and exclude inappropriate prescriptions
Assessment for oral corticosteroid therapy	Justify need for long-term treatment or supervise withdrawal
Bullous lung disease	Identify candidates for surgery
A rapid decline in FEV_1	Encourage early intervention
Assessment for pulmonary rehabilitation	Identify candidates for pulmonary rehabilitation
Assessment for lung volume reduction surgery	Identify candidates for surgery
Assessment for lung transplantation	Identify candidates for surgery
Dysfunctional breathing	Confirm diagnosis, optimise pharmacotherapy and access other therapists (e.g. physiotherapist)
Onset of symptoms under 40 years or a family history of alpha 1-antitrypsin deficiency	Identify alpha1-antitrypsin deficiency, consider therapy and screen family
Uncertain diagnosis	Make a diagnosis
Symptoms disproportionate to lung function deficit	Look for other explanations including cardiac impairment, pulmonary hypertension, depression and hyperventilation
Frequent infections	Exclude bronchiectasis
Haemoptysis	Exclude carcinoma of the bronchus

Table 12.3 Details of Primary Care review and follow up

Mild/moderate/severe (stages 1 to 3)		Very severe (stage 4)
Frequency	At least annual	At least twice per year
Clinical assessment	smoking status and desire to quit adequacy of symptom control: - breathlessness - exercise tolerance - estimated exacerbation frequency presence of complications effects of each drug treatment inhaler technique need for referral to specialist and therapy services need for pulmonary rehabilitation	smoking status and desire to quit adequacy of symptom control: - breathlessness - exercise tolerance - estimated exacerbation frequency presence of cor pulmonale need for long-term oxygen therapy patient's nutritional state presence of depression effects of each drug treatment inhaler technique need for social services and occupational therapy input need for referral to specialist and therapy services need for pulmonary rehabilitation
Measurements to make	FEV_1 and FVC calculate BMI MRC dyspnoea score	FEV_1 and FVC calculate BMI MRC dyspnoea score SaO_2

Reference

National Clinical Guideline Centre (2010) Chronic obstructive pulmonary disease: the management of chronic obstructive pulmonary disease in adults in primary and secondary care. London. CG101. Available at http://guidance.nice.org.uk/CG101/ Guidance/pdf/English

THE GOLD GUIDELINES

What is GOLD?

GOLD is the Global Initiative for Chronic Obstructive Lung Disease – a world-wide strategy for the diagnosis, management and prevention of COPD. The guidelines were produced by an international panel of experts who methodically reviewed the known published scientific literature to produce a set of evidence-based guidance on what is known and, in many cases, not known about the pathogenesis and management of COPD. They were last updated in 2009.

The aim of these guidelines is to bring COPD and its care to the attention of governments, public health officials, healthcare workers and the general public in as many countries around the world as possible, particularly in the developing nations.

The GOLD definition of COPD

COPD is a preventable and treatable disease with some significant extra-pulmonary effects that may contribute to the severity in individual patients. Its pulmonary component is characterised by airflow limitation that is not fully reversible. The airflow limitation is usually progressive and associated with an abnormal inflammatory response of the lung to noxious particles or gases.

Main clinical indicators for considering a diagnosis of COPD

The main indicators of COPD are as follows:

- Dyspnoea that is:
  - progressive, worsening with time
  - persistent, being present every day
  - worse with exercise and during respiratory infections.
- Chronic cough: intermittent or every day; often present throughout the day but seldom only at night.
- Chronic sputum production: any pattern can indicate COPD.

- Acute bronchitis – repeated episodes.

- History of exposure to risk factors, especially tobacco smoke; also to occupational dusts and chemicals, and smoke from home cooking and heating fuel. Biomass fuels are seen as the most important cause of COPD in developing countries, particularly the Indian sub-continent, China and Central and South America, and this especially affects women.

The diagnosis should be confirmed by spirometry.

Classification of COPD by severity

There is now a uniformity of COPD severity staging based on spirometry that is common to all the world's major guidelines (Table 12.4). GOLD used to include an 'At Risk' group who had cough or sputum but normal spirometry. This was dropped as there was no evidence that they significantly progress to stage 1 COPD. However, this does not mean that patients with persistent cough or sputum should not be properly evaluated and given advice on such risks as smoking.

The prime indicator is FEV_1/FVC ratio, which if below 0.7 suggests airflow obstruction. Lung function parameters should be taken post bronchodilator.

Table 12.4 GOLD classification of COPD severity by spirometry

Severity stage	Spirometry levels	Characteristics
Mild	FEV_1/FVC <0.7 FEV_1 >80% predicted	Patient occasionally may have cough or breathlessness. Often unaware of any abnormality
Moderate	FEV_1/FVC <0.7 FEV_1 50–80% predicted	Usually some shortness of breath on exertion. Often present at this stage. May have exacerbations.
Severe	FEV_1/FVC < 0.7 FEV_1 30–50% predicted	Greater breathlessness, reduced exercise capacity and repeated exacerbations. Impaired life quality
Very severe	FEV_1/FVC <0.7 FEV_1 below 30% predicted	Severe disabling symptoms and frequent exacerbations. Also included are patients with respiratory failure who have an FEV_1 >50% predicted

Goals of management

The goals of COPD management are to:

- prevent disease progression
- relieve symptoms
- improve exercise tolerance
- improve health status
- prevent and treat complications of COPD
- prevent and treat exacerbations
- prevent and minimise side-effects of treatment
- reduce mortality.

Assessing and monitoring disease

A detailed history in a new patient thought to have COPD should assess:

- Exposure to risk factors, including intensity and duration
- Past medical history including asthma, allergy, sinusitis and nasal polyps, respiratory infections in childhood and other respiratory diseases
- Family history of COPD or other respiratory diseases
- Pattern of symptom development
- History of exacerbations or previous hospitalisations for respiratory disorders
- Presence of co-morbidities, such as heart failure, malignancies, osteoporosis, and musculoskeletal disorders which may also contribute to disability
- Appropriateness of current medical treatments
- Impact of disease on patient's life, including limitation of activity; missed work and economic impact; effect on family routines; and feelings of depression and anxiety

- Social and family support available to the patient
- Possibilities for reducing risk factors, especially smoking.

Physical examination is important, but it is rarely diagnostic and has low sensitivity.

Bronchodilator reversibility testing is useful to rule out a diagnosis of asthma, particularly in patients with an atypical history, e.g. asthma in childhood or symptoms that suggest asthma. The criteria for a significant change according to GOLD are **an increase in FEV_1 of more than 12% and an increase of more than 200ml above baseline**. These figures are different from those used in the UK where both COPD and asthma guidelines agree that a change of more than 400ml in FEV_1 is suggestive of asthma. The UK criteria seem to provide a more sensible level as over 50% of patients in the UPLIFT trial, although clinically confirmed to have COPD, when given salbutamol and ipratropium combined pre-trial improved by more than 200ml.

Other tests

Chest X-ray is not usually helpful in diagnosing COPD but is useful to exclude other diagnoses such as lung cancer, TB and heart failure.

Alpha-1 antitrypsin deficiency screening should be performed when COPD is diagnosed in patients of Caucasian descent under 45 years, or with a strong family history of COPD.

Managing stable COPD

The general principles very much mirror those in NICE, with disease severity assessed on a raft of clinical measures and not just airflow obstruction. Patient education can improve a variety of measures to help patients cope better with their illness.

Treatment is based on a stepwise treatment plan that reflects the symptoms and disease severity. Awareness of co-morbidities is emphasised. The same range of therapies are used to prevent exacerbations as in NICE.

Pharmacological therapy and pulmonary rehabilitation are similar to NICE. Management of exacerbations is also similar.

References

Pauwels R, Buist AS, Calverley PMA, et al. (2001) Global strategy for the diagnosis, management and prevention of COPD. *American Journal of Respiratory and Critical Care Medicine* **163**: 1256–76
The updated GOLD Guidelines – last version produced in 2009 – are to be found online only at www.goldcopd.com.

THE NATIONAL CLINICAL STRATEGY FOR COPD 2010

Consultation on a strategy for services for COPD in England

This document, produced by the Department of Health in England, was published for consultation in 2010. It sets out to define the process of best care and the services that need to be set up for patients with all stages of COPD, from those still asymptomatic to those at the end of life. It identifies strategies to educate the public about good lung health and target prevention of disease. It most importantly describes steps of personalised quality care for all patients with COPD.

At the time of writing this update to 'COPD in Primary Care' this is still a consultation document and has not been officially ratified by the Government. However, meetings are taking place around the country to promote its messages and ideals.

Aims of the strategy

The aims of the strategy are to advise how local communities can:

- prevent people getting COPD

- understand the risks of having poor lung health

- secure improvements to the diagnosis and care of people with the disease

- reduce health inequalities.

Practical advice and education on managing their disease should be available to support people with COPD, and their carers. High-quality health care and social support should be available to all patients. These measures should be effective and give value for money for tax payers.

Strategy objectives

The strategy covers six main objectives:

1 **Prevention** – people should be able to make healthy choices about their life and social habits and so reduce the risk of getting lung disease. In the main this centres on support for smoking cessation and other risk-reducing behaviour.

2 **Supporting early identification** – ensuring that people have more information on the symptoms of lung disease and encouraging them to seek advice from health professionals earlier. Just under 1 million patients in the UK have been diagnosed with COPD but it is estimated that the true number is nearer to 3 million. Identification of the 'missing millions' is a large area of work that will involve careful consideration of the best screening methods.

3 **Good quality early diagnosis** – patients should be able to obtain an accurate, quality-assured diagnosis (particularly spirometry) with clear differentiation of COPD from asthma and other diseases. When diagnosed, patients should get good quality information on the illness and services available, both on diagnosis and throughout the course of their care.

4 **High-quality care and support following diagnosis** – by developing an organised, proactive, multidisciplinary approach to the management of both chronic and acute care.

5 **Improving access to high-quality end-of-life care services**.

6 **Differentiation of asthma** – a chapter on asthma helps to examine differences between COPD and asthma and summarises good asthma management, as set out in current asthma guidelines.

Implementation

A key area of the document is how the best practice ideas are to be advertised to all levels of the Health Service and then converted to standard good practice. There is no new NHS money attached to the strategy and, with the need to generate large financial savings for years ahead, it is difficult to see how major programmes such as screening will be progressed. However, this is a long-term plan.

Key initial changes that are currently workable are:

- reviewing those people who are on both asthma and COPD registers

- reviewing home oxygen registers

- reducing hospital admissions

- reducing the length of hospital stay for patients with COPD, where possible

- developing better models of chronic disease management, with regular reviews, use of self-management plans and treatment to prevent exacerbations

- reducing admission rates for asthma.

Longer term aims will be focused on trying to prevent COPD and detecting mild stages of disease earlier.

Prevention and identification

As shown in Figure 12.1, the goal is to provide information to reduce the numbers of people developing COPD, and if they do, to identify them earlier so measures can be suggested to prevent disease progression. In the UK this means trying to discourage people from smoking and also reducing risks in the workplace.

Recommendations on measures on which to focus include:

- identifying local areas where COPD prevalence and risk is high (usually localities of high socio-economic deprivation, where smoking prevalence is high and diet poor), and planning more intensive interventions there

■ trying to educate the population about good lung health, including the risks of exposure to tobacco smoke and early symptoms of disease.

A case finding approach to identifying early disease may be the most staff and cost effective.

One of the hurdles to better understanding and knowledge of COPD is that, despite this being a common disease, only a small percentage of the population have heard of it as COPD. Most people have heard of chronic bronchitis and emphysema. There is also a reluctance on the part of the public to present to primary care when symptoms such as cough or breathlessness develop, as they are perceived as being related to smoking.

The strategy has identified groups of high-risk people for initial identification and prevention. These include male and female manual workers, people employed in industries exposed to dust and fumes, pregnant women who smoke, parents who smoke – risk to children and making children more likely to smoke – young children, older smokers (over 55 years) and Bangladeshi men.

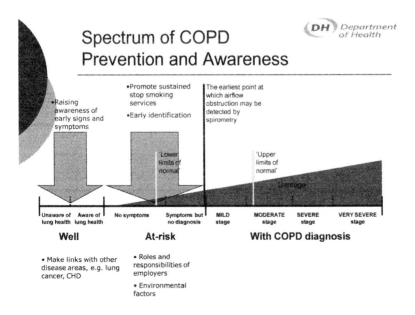

Figure 12.1 The National Clinical Strategy – Prevention and awareness

Finding the 'missing millions'

An estimated 2 million people have undiagnosed COPD, most of whom have mild or moderate disease. Early diagnosis and intervention may prevent disease progression.

The strategy recommends that healthcare professionals should understand the risk factors for COPD and offer appropriate advice or an intervention to those at risk.

In children there are a number of risk factors to be aware of – alpha-1 antitrypsin deficiency, maternal smoking in pregnancy, premature or small babies, severe respiratory infections and asthma in early childhood, environmental tobacco smoke and smoking in early childhood. As a result of some of these, children will have impaired lung function in the first decade of life and a potential screening opportunity might be performing spirometry at the age of 14 years. Offering specific advice at this age, particularly about smoking, may prevent disease.

In adults the main risk factors are smoking and occupational exposure. A case finding programme using specific symptom questionnaires and spirometry is being considered. People over 40 with respiratory symptoms or risk factors should be screened.

Quality assured spirometry

A key recommendation is that the diagnosis of COPD should be confirmed by quality assured spirometry, and other investigations appropriate to the individual. The strategy stresses the importance of good spirometric technique, based on an accredited training course, and maintaining equipment. Standards of training and spirometric performance are currently inadequate.

Classification of severity

The GOLD classification of airflow obstruction severity has also been adopted by the strategy with the same provisos regarding patients with stage 1 disease who are asymptomatic. Similar points are made about overestimation of disease using the FEV_1/FVC ratio in older patients. They agree that using the LLN 5% would be more accurate and await better reference tables before adopting this change.

High quality care and support

The spectrum of chronic care is outlined in Figure 12.2.

Recording relevant data

Severity of COPD is assessed, as in the NICE update, by assessing other clinical parameters such as MRC Dyspnoea score and exacerbations, as well as spirometry.

Better recording of relevant data on the GP disease register will provide better and more accurate information on the patient. The following ought to be recorded:

- actual FEV_1, whether pre or post bronchodilator and severity grade of the new NICE criteria

- symptoms such as cough, sputum and breathlessness

- functional impairment such as MRC Dyspnoea

- exacerbation frequency

- BMI

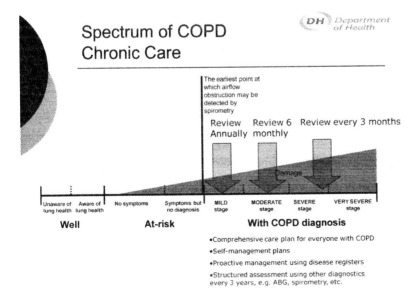

Figure 12.2 National Clinical Strategy – Chronic care

- smoking history and current status
- oxygen assessment
- educational knowledge of COPD
- co-morbidities including psychological status, cardiovascular disease, diabetes and osteoporosis
- ethnic group
- wishes for palliative and end-of-life care when identification of advanced disease has occurred.

Information for patients

The strategy recommends that good quality information about COPD should be provided at diagnosis, in a format that any patient can understand. In workshops with COPD patients the areas that patients most required information were:

- education about the disease
- management of breathlessness
- pharmacological treatments
- managing exacerbations
- psychological support
- guidance on welfare benefits.

Management

Treatment follows the guidelines set out in the NICE update and other sections of this book.

In summary, COPD patients should have an integrated chronic disease management approach, irrespective of disease severity. Regular structured reviews are a key part of this process. Self-management and interaction with any other health professionals and others with COPD able to provide information and advice should be encouraged. Management of exacerbations should be improved and every effort made to reduce the frequency of future exacerbations. All people with respiratory failure should be given oxygen alert cards and ambulance staff should be able to respond to these when involved.

End-of-life care

People with COPD have far less palliative care than patients with cancer, despite the number of annual deaths from COPD and lung cancer being comparable. The main reasons for this are that it is often clinically difficult to give an accurate prognosis for COPD patients and to tell when patients are entering their final six months of life. Also, until recently, there was little provision of palliative care for conditions that were not cancer.

As we have discussed in Chapter 10, the disease trajectories towards death for cancer and COPD are very different (see Figures 10.1 and 10.2). Cancer changes over a relatively short period of rapid decline before death – often only a few weeks. COPD generally deteriorates slowly over years with frequent exacerbations, although any one of them may cause death. The systematic use of The Gold Standards Framework and the compilation of registers of patients likely to need palliative care support, as supported by the General Medical Services Contract QOF, provide a good starting point towards identifying those individuals with COPD who may benefit from palliative services.

The strategy supports better access to high quality palliative care services. There should also be ready access to information and support for carers and those bereaved.

As mentioned, it is often difficult to determine the period of need for extra end-of-life care in COPD. A number of markers may be helpful:

- severe airflow obstruction with FEV_1 below 30% predicted

- respiratory failure

- low BMI – below 19

- housebound

- two or more admissions with exacerbations in previous year

- need for non-invasive ventilation (NIV) for acute exacerbation.

There should be access to a full range of supportive care which addresses symptoms, pain, anxiety and depression, cachexia and fatigue, home oxygen, social support, advanced care planning, etc. as required

Further information

Copies of the National Strategy are available to order online at www.orderline.dh.gov.uk quoting 296481/Consultation on a Strategy for Services for Chronic Obstructive Pulmonary Disease (COPD) in England.

THE NICE QUALITY STANDARDS FOR COPD

NICE in conjunction with the Department of Health are currently producing a range of Quality Standards that summarise best practice for COPD and many other chronic diseases. The COPD quality standards are, at the time of writing, in draft form and are out for consultation. The anticipated publication date is June 2011. These standards will be applicable to all levels of the NHS and stress the need for an integrated approach for provision of services.

There are 13 quality statements.

1 People receiving a clinical diagnosis of COPD have a record of one or more indicative presenting symptoms.

2 People with COPD have their diagnosis confirmed by post-bronchodilator spirometry carried out by health professionals competent in its performance and interpretation.

3 People with COPD have a comprehensive assessment of severity that includes the degree of breathlessness, the frequency of exacerbations and an evaluation of health status using a validated measure.

4 People with COPD who smoke are encouraged to stop and offered help to do so.

5 People with COPD are offered inhaled therapies in accordance with NICE guidance.

6 People with COPD who are prescribed oxygen therapy are assessed in accordance with NICE guidance.

7 People with COPD who are prescribed oxygen are clinically assessed and have their oxygen therapy reviewed at least once a year.

8 People with COPD, meeting appropriate criteria, are offered an effective pulmonary rehabilitation programme.

9 People who have had an exacerbation of COPD are given self-management advice and a course of antibiotic and corticosteroid tablets to keep at home.

10 People with COPD, an exacerbation of COPD and persistent acidotic ventilatory failure are offered non–invasive ventilation delivered by trained staff in a dedicated setting.

11 People with COPD admitted to hospital because of an exacerbation have access to an assisted discharge scheme.

12 People with advanced COPD, and their carers, have access to specialist palliative care services if required.

13 People diagnosed with COPD receive written and verbal information about their condition and its management.

13 | Organisation and training needs

Main points

1 Primary care will have a major role in achieving the objectives of the National Clinical Strategy for COPD and raising the standards of care.

2 Structured primary care management may result in:

- fewer emergency consultations
- improved understanding and self-management skills for patients
- rational use of medication.

3 Strategies to identify individuals with undiagnosed COPD, together with reappraisal of the practice asthma register to reveal patients who have COPD rather than asthma, are needed to identify the 'missing millions' of COPD patients.

4 Spirometry is crucial for the accurate and early detection of COPD, but needs to be performed and interpreted by adequately trained personnel and, ideally, quality assured. Which model of spirometry service provision is most appropriate needs to be decided at local level, and depends on local circumstances.

6 Nurses can provide good structured care for COPD patients but the level of their involvement must depend on their training. GP support and good communication between all members of the primary healthcare team is essential.

7 Audit of the outcomes of COPD care is necessary to the continuing development of good standards of care.

8 The UK General Medical Services contract Quality Outcomes Framework allows for payment to general practices who have achieved to following quality standards:

- The practice can produce a register of COPD patients,
- 40–80% of patients diagnosed after 1 April 2008 have

had their diagnosis confirmed by post-bronchodilator spirometry

- 40–70% of the patients on the COPD register have had their FEV_1 recorded in the previous 15 months
- 50–90% of the patients have been reviewed by a healthcare professional in the past 15 months, including an assessment of breathlessness using the MRC dyspnoea score
- 40–85% of the patients have been immunised against influenza in the previous period, 1 September to 31 March

In an average GP list of 2,500 patients there are likely to be between 550 and 600 smokers (given an average smoking rate of about 23%), of whom around 100–150 are likely to have COPD. In areas of social deprivation, where smoking rates are higher and where the population is exposed to a greater number of risk factors, such as occupational exposures, crowded, substandard housing and poor nutrition, this number will be higher. Many of these patients will not be known to their doctor, because they will have mild to moderate disease – so they will be undiagnosed and untreated. On the other hand, many of those whose disease has progressed will be presenting with recurrent chest infections and some will have been misdiagnosed as suffering from asthma. Those who have severe COPD are likely to be attending hospital and to have been admitted several times with exacerbations of their disease.

Structured asthma management clinics in primary care are now commonplace and it is often the practice nurse who plays a major role. COPD patients may have referred themselves to the practice asthma clinic, hoping for a new approach; or the GP will have referred them, having run out of ideas about what to do for these 'heart sink' patients. However, a focus on asthma and a lack of training in COPD may lead to patients with COPD being treated inappropriately along asthma management guidelines, and effective COPD therapies, pharmacological and non-pharmacological, not being considered.

In the past there were no guidelines as to how patients with COPD should be managed, and little training for primary care physicians and nurses. Management tended to be of the 'crisis intervention' variety and there was little understanding of the concepts of proper assessment, diagnosis or long-term management goals for COPD. Contrary to previously held beliefs, we now know that there are interventions that can improve the quality of life of people with COPD and that have potential to reduce the burden the disease places on individuals and their families, the health service and society as a whole.

A resurgence of interest in COPD, training opportunities for healthcare professionals, the publication of evidence-based guidelines from NICE and GOLD and the added incentive of payment for providing care for COPD patients in primary care under the General Medical Service contract is stimulating improvement in the care these patients receive. The National Clinical Strategy aims to enhance further best care, ensuring equitable access to high-quality services and reducing the current high cost of unscheduled care for this debilitating condition.

The main objectives of the consultation document on the National Clinical Strategy are discussed in detail in the previous chapter. Clearly, primary care has a major role in reaching these objectives. Proper diagnosis and management in primary care should result in patients being diagnosed earlier and managed better – and will, hopefully, result in fewer of them being referred for specialist care and repeatedly admitted to hospital.

Finding the patients

The 'missing millions'

It is estimated that there are at least 2 million individuals in England and Wales who have undiagnosed COPD. Identifying these individuals, so that they can be treated and managed appropriately to reduce disease progression and lessen disability, is the first objective of the National Clinical Strategy.

Primary care healthcare professionals already collect data on smoking status and are well placed to discover other risk factors for COPD in the people registered with them and to raise general awareness of COPD. Primary care is also the first port of call for patients with early symptoms. A systematic approach to screening and offering advice and support to those at risk of COPD will go some way to reaching the first objective of the National Clinical Strategy.

Re-evaluation of the asthma register

Patients with advanced COPD are likely to be known to you, but it is also probable that there are some with moderate disease who have been given an incorrect diagnostic label and are being managed inappropriately. A good starting point, therefore, is to re-examine the practice asthma register, looking particularly at patients over 35 years of age with a current or previous smoking history and who are taking asthma medication. A reassessment of each patient's records and reappraisal of how the diagnosis of asthma was reached may reveal those whose history is more in keeping with a diagnosis of COPD than asthma and those in whom an objective, 'water-tight' diagnosis of asthma is lacking. A synopsis of the features of COPD compared with those of asthma is given in Table 13.1.

The next step is to evaluate the patient's spirometry. If the spirometry is obstructed and the history is consistent with COPD rather than asthma, the patient's therapy may need to be re-evaluated.

Table 13.1 A comparison of the features of COPD and asthma

	COPD	*Asthma*
Onset of symptoms	**Aged 35+ years**	Aged +/– 35 years, 'childhood chestiness' (with or without history of atopic illness)
Smoking history	**15–20+ pack-years**	No or light smoking history
Family history	With or without a history of 'emphysema' 'Chronic bronchitis'	Atopic illness/asthma
Symptoms	**Non-variable Shortness of breath on exertion,** cough and sputum with or without wheeze, 'chest tightness'	**Variable** Wheeze, 'chest tightness', cough and sputum in exacerbations
Nocturnal wakening	Rare	**Common**
Morning symptoms	Rapidly relieved by expectoration	Last several hours
Response to asthma medication	Moderate at best	Usually good

The features in **bold** are the particularly relevant ones.

The area of pharmacotherapy most fruitful to examine is the use of bronchodilators, particularly the antimuscarinics. A trial of these agents may produce additional symptomatic benefit. The patient's educational needs and the use of other non-pharmacological therapies, such as pulmonary rehabilitation, may also need to be considered.

Most of the patients from the asthma register who are being re-evaluated to see if they actually have COPD will already be taking inhaled corticosteroids. All major guidelines now recommend the use of high dose inhaled corticosteroids in all patients with moderate to severe disease (FEV_1 less than 50% predicted) who suffer two or more exacerbations a year, requiring treatment with antibiotics or oral corticosteroids. The NICE 2010 update has extended this recommendation to include those with less severe airflow obstruction and frequent exacerbations or uncontrolled symptoms. Formal corticosteroid trials are therefore not usually indicated for these patients, and are often unhelpful. It may, however, be worthwhile reviewing the dose of inhaled corticosteroids being used as it may need increasing in a patient with COPD rather than asthma. Since inhaled corticosteroids as a solo agent are not licensed for COPD it is recommended they be given as a combined inhaler with a long acting bronchodilator – LABA.

In the few cases where it is suspected that high-dose inhaled corticosteroids are being given inappropriately consideration can be given to slow reduction of the dose, as follows:

- Reduce the dose by 25% every three months.

- Review the patient frequently, observing for rapidly declining lung function or deterioration of symptoms.

This approach, whilst not giving rapid results, would seem logical. If a patient with asthma is already optimally controlled on inhaled corticosteroids, any response to an oral corticosteroid trial is likely to be masked, giving a false-negative result. The inhaled corticosteroids may then be discontinued when they are needed. The slow reduction of inhaled corticosteroids is also supported by an observational report from the Isolde COPD trial. When these were abruptly withdrawn from patients in the seven-week run-in period to the trial, 32% of the patients suffered an exacerbation.

Case-finding and screening

Reappraisal of the practice asthma register may improve the diagnosis rate in patients with moderate to severe disease and allow more rational prescribing and patient management, but it is unlikely to improve the diagnosis rate in patients with mild, largely asymptomatic, disease and those with mild to moderate disease who may be attending with 'chest infections' in the winter. It is an unfortunate fact that, by the time symptoms of COPD become apparent, considerable and irreversible loss of lung function has already occurred. If severe, debilitating, expensive and life-threatening disease is to be prevented, it must be detected early and smoking cessation advice and support given. If awareness of the possibility of COPD is raised with smokers who attend with occasional 'chest infections' and they are screened with spirometry, the detection rate for early COPD is likely to improve.

A case-finding approach and the use of questionnaires to detect suitable candidates for spirometry has already been discussed in Chapter 4; those with symptoms, i.e. chronic cough, sputum, breathlessness and/or exercise limitation. Whilst the value of screening completely asymptomatic smokers remains controversial the National Clinical Strategy has identified a number of groups that could be considered to be particularly at risk and suitable for case finding and spirometry:

- ex-smokers

- people with a previous history of pulmonary tuberculosis

- first-degree relatives of patients with COPD

- people who have had a known occupational exposure

- those with chronic asthma

- individuals who have required frequent courses of antibiotics for lower respiratory tract infections and/or inhaled medication

- people with a known environmental exposure (e.g. coal mining, those from abroad exposed to wood-burning stoves).

The strategy suggests that priority be given to those at most risk; smokers and ex-smokers with 20 or more 'pack years' who are aged over 40, those who have been treated with frequent courses of antibiotics and/or inhaled medication or those with symptoms such as chronic cough or breathlessness.

Spirometry

The role of spirometry in the detection and diagnosis of COPD has already been discussed. However, spirometers are expensive and they must be used properly if the results are not to be meaningless. Incorrectly performed spirometry may result in patients being referred for specialist opinion unnecessarily, or patients needing referral being missed. The need for good, quality assured spirometry is stressed in The National Clinical Strategy. Training in the correct use and care of equipment and in interpretation of the results is essential. The proposed standards document for primary care spirometry, published in 2009, recommends that training be subject to assessment of competence in both performance and interpretation of spirometry.

A machine that complies with European and American Guidelines for lung function testing and the proposed standards for spirometry in primary care, together with providing the necessary training, is likely to cost in excess of £1,500. The spirometer also needs to be used often enough to maintain the skills of the operator, once they have achieved competence. This may not be practicable for every general practice. The various models of service delivery for spirometry are discussed in Chapter 5 and are covered in detail in the proposed standards document. Which of these options is most practical must be decided at a local level.

The practice nurse's role

Throughout this book we have emphasised the need for a structured approach to diagnosis and management and the need for patient education, involving both the GP and the practice nurse. This is also the focus of the second and third objectives of the National Clinical Strategy. The effectiveness of this approach with asthma patients has been widely studied and its benefits well established, but there remains a dearth of research relating to COPD. However, it would seem logical that COPD patients will benefit from a similar approach and it is recommended in the NICE guideline and rewarded under the Quality Outcomes Framework. The fact that COPD and asthma differ has also been emphasised in this book, to stress how important it is that health professionals caring for patients have a sound understanding of those differences and their implications for treatment.

Providing a structured approach to care in COPD requires doctor or nurse time. In practices already running asthma clinics, extending the scope of the clinic to include COPD management – an 'airways clinic' – is one possible approach. Many COPD patients attend 'asthma clinics', so this may be a practicable option.

Appropriately trained nurses have had – and continue to have – a major impact on asthma management. How involved GPs and nurses are in COPD management should depend on their knowledge, interest and expertise. Whatever their role, they must be trained for it and should have been assessed as competent. The routine care of asthma patients has, in many practices, been almost completely devolved to nurses. However, COPD patients are usually older, often have multiple pathologies and can be more difficult to manage. They are a group of patients for whom a team approach is essential. Appropriately trained nurses can develop a great deal of expertise in COPD, but may be relatively inexperienced in the management of, for example, ischaemic heart disease, so it is vital that they recognise their limitations (Table 13.2). Easy communication between members of the team and appreciation of each other's expertise and role are essential.

Protocol and audit

It is necessary to have a practice protocol that clearly defines how patients are managed and describes the roles of each member of the primary care team in place from the outset. Thought needs to be given as to whether nurses involved need to be prescribers, or whether patient group directions that allow the nurse to carry out reversibility testing are needed. (If the GP does not prescribe the drugs for each individual needing a reversibility test, and the nurse is not a prescriber, patient group directions for this situation are a legal requirement.) The protocol should be agreed and followed by all members of the team so that the approach is systematic and logical, and patients receive consistent advice. It should follow current guidelines for the care of COPD. Suggestions for what should be considered when formulating a practice protocol are given in Table 13.3.

Table 13.2 The role of the practice nurse

Minimum involvement

Maintain a register of known COPD patients

Call COPD patients annually for influenza vaccination

Ensure that COPD patients have received pneumococcal vaccination

Encourage patients to stop smoking, and advise them at each visit

Teach and check inhaler technique

Provide information to patients and their relatives about COPD – e.g. British Lung Foundation

(The patient is managed and followed up by the GP)

Suggested training:

In-house training

Local study evenings in COPD and smoking cessation

Basic COPD course – e.g. Education for Health COPD Short Course

Basic smoking cessation course – e.g. Education for Health Smoking Cessation Short Course

+ EXPERIENCE

Medium involvement

As for 'Minimum involvement', plus:

Take a basic respiratory history

Carry out diagnostic procedures – e.g. spirometry and reversibility testing – when indicated

Update the COPD register

Establish a regular follow-up procedure for COPD patients

Provide basic information and advice on diet and exercise

(The patient is cared for jointly by the GP and the practice nurse)

Training needs:

Spirometry training: caring for the equipment, getting a technically acceptable result and basic interpretation – e.g. Education for Health diploma level Spirometry Module. Successful candidates also receive the ARTP Certificate of Competence in Spirometry

Assessed diploma level training in COPD – e.g. Education for Health COPD Module

+ EXPERIENCE

Maximum involvement

As for 'Medium involvement', plus:

Take a full respiratory history

Perform a basic examination of the patient to assess for hyperinflation, central cyanosis and oedema

Be able to recognise abnormal spirometry

Suggest further investigation – chest X-ray, ECG, full blood count, etc.

Assess disability and handicap

Instigate therapeutic trials and evaluate their effectiveness

Assess the need for pulmonary rehabilitation and refer/instigate as necessary

Advise patients on self-management

Liaise with other appropriate health professionals

Provide regular follow-up and support for patients and their families

(The patient is managed and followed up by the nurse, with GP support and advice)

Training needs:

Spirometry interpretation course – e.g. ARTP certification or Education for Health degree level Spirometry Module

Assessed degree-level training in COPD – e.g. Education for Health Advanced COPD Module

Assessed degree-level training in assessing patients with undiagnosed cardiorespiratory symptoms – e.g. Education for Health Cardiorespiratory Symptoms: assessment and diagnosis.

The effectiveness of your practice's COPD management should be audited, so that standards can be maintained and improved, and any deficiencies highlighted and remedied. There has been little research to determine which outcome measures should be audited, but the draft NICE Quality Standards discussed in the previous chapter provide markers of good quality care, against which to examine and improve your own service. The suggestions listed in Table 13.4 include General Medical Service contract performance indicators and NICE recommendations.

For the health professional the proper management of COPD patients can be immensely rewarding and satisfying. Many patients have been dismissed as 'hopeless cases'. They frequently have low

Table 13.3 Example of a practice protocol

Case finding and maintenance of disease register
- Update diagnosis opportunistically
- Opportunistic and new patient screening
- Systematic search of patient records (aged 40+, recurrent 'chest infection', smoker)
- Reappraisal of practice asthma register

Diagnostic criteria
- Symptoms
- Lung function – post-bronchodilator spirometry essential
- Reversibility to bronchodilators and corticosteroids, when indicated
- Other investigations – chest x-ray, ECG, full blood count, etc.

Treatment
- Disease severity recorded
- Response to therapeutic bronchodilator trials measured objectively and recorded
- Stepwise approach to drug treatment

Referral criteria
- Referral for specialist opinion
- Referral for admission during exacerbation
- Referral for pulmonary rehabilitation

Follow-up and recall
- Review and recall of patients on practice register
- Annual review of patients – to include:
  - functional status
  - general health status – e.g. measured with the CAT score
  - BMI
  - MRC dyspnoea score
  - assessment for anxiety and depression
  - response to therapy
  - exacerbation rate in previous 12 months
  - FEV_1 in patients with rapidly declining functional status or frequent exacerbation
  - pulse oximetry if FEV_1 less than 50% predicted
  - review of management.
- Follow-up of patients admitted to hospital
- Review of patients on long-term oxygen and nebulisers

Smoking cessation policy
- Record smoking status and 'tag' patient records
- Discuss and encourage the use of nicotine replacement therapy, bupropion or varenicline
- Referral of patients to smoking cessation services, or review and recall patients who are 'quitting'

Table 13.3 Example of a practice protocol

Delegation of care and internal referral policy
- Named GP with overall responsibility
- Role of practice nurse (according to expertise and training)
- Role of support staff

Table 13.4 COPD audit

Audit of process
Percentage of smokers who have had spirometry performed
Number of patients on the COPD register
Number of newly diagnosed patients who have had the diagnosis
confirmed by post-bronchodilator spirometry and have one or more
clinical indicators of COPD
Number of patients who were ever diagnosed by spirometry
Number of patients still smoking
Number who have had smoking cessation advice
Number of smokers referred to the local specialist smoking cessation
service
In the previous year:
Number who have had FEV_1 recorded
Number who have had their inhaler technique checked
Number who have a record of BMI
Number who have a record of MRC dyspnoea score
Number who have a record of exacerbation frequency
Number who have had an evaluation of health status (e.g. CAT score)
Number who have been assessed for depression, using the standard
screening questions
Number of patients with severe and very severe COPD who have had an
oxygen saturation recorded
Number of those who have had an exacerbation and been given written
self-management advice
Number of those who have had an exacerbation and been prescribed
stand-by courses of oral steroids and/or antibiotics
Number who have had influenza vaccine in the previous season
Number vaccinated against pneumococcus

Audit of outcome
Number of patients still smoking
Number of emergency admissions
Number of emergency GP consultations
Disability scores
Handicap scores
Percentage of those with MRC dyspnoea score of 3 or more referred for
pulmonary rehabilitation.

---

self-esteem and poor expectations. Trevor Clay OBE – former Secretary of the Royal College of Nursing (RCN), tireless campaigner for the British Lung Foundation Breathe Easy groups and a COPD sufferer – summed up the problems many COPD patients face when he addressed the RCN Respiratory Nurses Forum:

'Our [Breathe Easy's] aim is to remove the phrase 'there's nothing more that can be done' from the vocabulary of health professionals. Not only does it have a devastating effect but it is simply not true. What is meant is that there is no magic, no cure, but there is always something that can be done.'

A greater awareness and understanding of COPD should improve the standard of care that COPD patients receive and should ultimately result in a reduction in the burden that this devastating disease causes.

Further reading

Department of Health (2010) Consultation on a strategy for services for Chronic Obstructive Pulmonary Disease (COPD) in England. Available at www.orderline.dh.gov.uk

Levy M, Quanjer PH, Booker R, et al. (2009) Diagnostic spirometry in primary care: proposed standards for general practice compliant with American Thoracic Society and European Respiratory Society recommendations. *Primary Care Respiratory Journal* **18** (3): 130-47

National Clinical Guideline Centre (2010) Chronic obstructive pulmonary disease: the management of chronic obstructive pulmonary disease in adults in primary and secondary care. London. CG101. Available at http://guidance.nice.org.uk/CG101/Guidance/pdf/English

Useful addresses

British Lung Foundation
73–75 Goswell Road
London EC1V 7ER
Tel: 020 7688 5555
Fax: 020 7688 5556
Website: www.lunguk.org

Education for Health
The Athenaeum
10 Church Street
Warwick CV34 4AB
Tel: 01926 493313
Fax: 01926 493224
Website: www.educationforhealth.org.uk

Glossary

Words shown in *italic* in the definition are also defined in this Glossary

ACE inhibitor angiotensin-converting enzyme inhibitor – a class of drugs used in hypertension and cardiac failure

adaptive aerosol delivery (AAD) an innovative nebuliser system that delivers drug during inhalation only and can be programmed to deliver a precise amount of drug

aerobic exercise exercise to increase the efficiency of the heart and lungs in delivering oxygen to the tissues

air-trapping excess air remaining in the lung at the end of exhalation. This may be due to airway collapse and/or loss of lung elasticity, as in *emphysema*

airway hyper-responsiveness the airways are over-reactive and 'irritable' and more likely to constrict in response to a wide variety of physical and chemical stimuli

alpha-1 antitrypsin ($\boxtimes_1$-AT) an *antiprotease* in the blood. Congenital deficiency of alpha-1 antitrypsin is associated with the early presentation (under 40 years of age) of severe *emphysema*

alveolar/capillary interface the surface of the lung where gas exchange occurs

anticholinergic bronchodilator a drug that inhibits the action of acetylcholine on parasympathetic nerve endings in the lungs and dilates airways

antioxidants substances that neutralise oxidants. They occur naturally in foods rich in vitamins C and E, and may help to slow the rate of progression of COPD

antiprotease/elastase enzyme that neutralises protease/elastase (enzymes that destroy lung tissue by digesting *elastin*, one of the proteins that makes up lung parenchyma)

251

arterial blood gases measurement of the amount of oxygen and carbon dioxide dissolved in the plasma of an arterial blood sample, measured in kilopascals (kPa)

asthma chronic inflammatory condition of the airways, leading to widespread, variable airway obstruction that is reversible spontaneously or with treatment. Long-standing asthma may become unresponsive to treatment

atopy hereditary predisposition to develop allergic *asthma*, rhinitis and eczema. It is associated with high levels of the antibody IgE

beta-2 agonist bronchodilator a drug that stimulates the betaadrenergic receptors in the lungs, resulting in bronchodilation

Blue Badge (formerly **Orange Badge**) **scheme** a scheme for disabled persons, allowing them to park in restricted areas

'blue bloater' a somewhat outmoded term used to describe a cyanosed COPD patient who is oedematous and at risk of *cor pulmonale*

Borg scale a measure of breathlessness by which the patient quantifies the amount of breathlessness that an activity produces

breath-assisted nebuliser a jet nebuliser that boosts output during inhalation and minimises drug wastage during exhalation

Breathe Easy Club the name of patient support groups facilitated by the British Lung Foundation

bronchiectasis irreversible dilation of the bronchi due to bronchial wall damage, causing chronic cough and mucopurulent sputum

broncho-alveolar lavage a technique used to wash samples of cells from small airways and alveoli. It is performed during bronchoscopy

bronchomotor tone the amount of bronchial muscle contraction (tone) normally present in the airways. This is often increased in COPD patients

bullous emphysema large cyst-like spaces in the lung that compress normal lung tissue. It may be amenable to surgery

chronic bronchitis sputum production that occurs on most days for at least three months in at least two consecutive years (Medical Research Council definition)

chronic obstructive pulmonary disease (COPD) a slowly progressive disorder characterised by airflow obstruction, which does not change markedly over several months (British Thoracic Society definition)

collagen a connective tissue. Deposition of collagen in the basement membrane of small airways contributes to irreversible airflow obstruction

cor pulmonale pulmonary hypertension and right ventricular hypertrophy (and eventual failure) occurring as a result of chronic lung disease. It causes peripheral oedema, raised jugular venous pressure and liver enlargement

corticosteroid reversibility a test done to determine which COPD patients have significant response (an increase in FEV_1 greater than 200ml and 15% of baseline) to steroids and who merit long-term inhaled steroids. Large improvements are indicative of *asthma* rather than COPD. Prednisolone 30mg is given in the morning for two weeks. Alternatively 1000µg per day of beclometasone (or equivalent) is given for six weeks

corticosteroids/steroids hormones produced by the adrenal glands. Synthetic forms are used in COPD for their anti-inflammatory activity, although their long-term use is controversial

cyanosis blueness of the skin due to hypoxia. It is a somewhat subjective finding but when oxygen saturation falls below 85–90% cyanosis generally becomes apparent

cyclic adenosine monophosphate (cyclic AMP) a substance found in cells that has a crucial role in bronchodilation and reduction of inflammation

cytokines glycoprotein molecules that regulate cell-to-cell communication of the inflammatory response

dynamic airway collapse the tendency of unsupported airways to collapse during forced exhalation

elastase enzyme that digests *elastin*

elastin protein that makes up lung tissue. Its elastic properties contribute to the lung's elastic recoil and helps expel air from the lungs during exhalation

emphysema abnormal permanent enlargement of the air spaces distal to the terminal bronchiole (alveoli) accompanied by destruction of their walls

eosinophil white blood cell. It is characteristically found in the airways of people with asthma and is implicated in long-term inflammation and epithelial damage

FEV_1 see *forced expired volume*

fibrosing alveolitis a condition resulting in widespread *fibrosis* of the alveoli. It causes progressive breathlessness and a restrictive spirometry pattern

fibrosis scarring and thickening of an organ or tissue by replacement of the original tissue with collagenous fibrous tissue

flow/volume trace a graph produced by a spirometer in which flow rate (in litres per second) is on the vertical axis and volume (in litres) on the horizontal axis

forced expired volume (FEV$_1$) the amount of air that can be exhaled in the first second of a forced blow from maximum inhalation

forced vital capacity (FVC) the total volume of air that can be exhaled from a maximal inhalation to maximal exhalation

gas transfer test (TLCO) a test performed in lung function laboratories that determines the ability of the lungs to take up a small amount of carbon monoxide. It is a measure of how efficiently the *alveolar/capillary interface* is working

'guy-rope effect' the support given to small airways by the elastic walls of the alveoli in the lung parenchyma

health status/quality of life a measure of the impact of a disease on a patient's daily life, and social and emotional well-being

Hoover's sign in-drawing of the lower intercostal margins on inhalation

hypercapnia high levels of carbon dioxide in the blood. Levels over 6kPa are generally considered to be abnormal

hypoxia low levels of oxygen in the blood. Levels below 10kPa are generally considered to be abnormal

hypoxic challenge a method of assessing the response of a patient to the reduced oxygen levels they will encounter during air travel

hypoxic respiratory drive a stimulus to breathe that is driven by low levels of oxygen. When patients with this abnormal drive are given high levels of oxygen the stimulus to breathe will be suppressed, resulting in worsening respiratory failure or respiratory arrest

immunoglobulin E (IgE) an antibody. Raised levels of IgE are associated with *atopy* and allergy

inhaled corticosteroids/steroids *corticosteroids* available as beclometasone, budesonide or fluticasone in a variety of inhaler devices

jet nebulisers the most commonly used nebuliser. Atomising the drug solution in the airflow from a compressor or piped gas supply produces the aerosol

leukotriene antagonists a new class of drugs for *asthma* that either block the formation of leukotrienes or block the leukotriene receptors in the lungs

long-term oxygen therapy (LTOT) oxygen given for 15 hours or more a day. It improves life expectancy and may improve health status in chronically hypoxic COPD patients

losartan a recently developed angiotensin II inhibitor that reduces pulmonary artery pressure in COPD

lung volume reduction surgery a new technique developed in the USA to remove 20–30% of the most emphysematous parts of the lung and improve breathlessness

lymphocytes white blood cells involved in the body's immune system

macrophages white blood cells that are involved in phagocytosis and secretion of cytokines that attract and activate neutrophils and other inflammatory cells

mast cells white blood cells that release histamine and other inflammatory mediators. *Immunoglobulin E* is attached to their surfaces

nicotine replacement therapy (NRT) a method of reducing craving and withdrawal symptoms in people attempting to stop smoking. It is available as chewing gum, transdermal patches, inhalator, nasal spray, lozenges and sublingual tablets. It can double success rates

obliterative bronchiolitis widespread fibrotic, inflammatory condition of the small airways. A late and serious complication of lung transplantation, it is frequently fatal in 6–12 months

obstructive sleep apnoea (OSA) upper airway obstruction occurring during sleep. It may result in repeated and significant episodes of hypoxia and severe sleep deprivation. Can cause *cor pulmonale* and may coexist with COPD. Commonly presents with daytime somnolence and a history of severe snoring

occupational asthma variable airway obstruction resulting from exposure to a sensitising agent inhaled at work. Continued exposure to the causative agent may result in severe, persistent asthma with irreversibility

osteoporosis demineralisation and atrophy of bone, associated with an increased risk of fracture. It is most commonly seen in post-menopausal women but is also associated with long-term use of oral corticosteroids

oxidants see *oxygen radicals/oxidants*

oxygen concentrator electrically powered molecular 'sieve' that removes nitrogen and carbon dioxide and delivers almost pure oxygen to the patient. It is a cost-effective method of delivering long-term oxygen

oxygen cost diagram a measure of disability in which a patient marks a 10cm line against an activity that induces breathlessness. The disability score is the distance along the line

oxygen radicals/oxidants highly active molecules – found in tobacco smoke and released by inflammatory cells – that can damage lung tissue

oxygen saturation the percentage of haemoglobin saturated with oxygen. It is measured with a pulse oximeter. Normal oxygen saturation is over 95%. Cyanosis is apparent with a saturation of between 85% and 90%

peak expiratory flow (PEF) the maximal flow rate that can be maintained over the first 10 milliseconds of a forced blow

phosphodiesterase inhibitors a group of drugs, including *theophyllines*, that increase *cyclic AMP* levels and may reduce inflammation and cause bronchodilation

photochemical pollutants gases such as ozone, produced by the action of sunlight on vehicle exhaust gases

'pink puffer' a somewhat outmoded term to describe a COPD patient who is very breathless but has normal arterial blood gases and is not at risk of the early development of *cor pulmonale*

pneumococcal vaccination recommended for COPD patients by the Department of Health although controlled studies of its effectiveness are lacking

pneumotachograph a device for measuring flow rates. Some electronic spirometers use these to assess flow rates and calculate lung volumes from the flow rates

polycythaemia an abnormal increase in the number of red blood cells. In COPD this can occur as a result of chronic *hypoxia*

pulmonary oedema extravasated fluid in the lung tissue. Commonly caused by left ventricular failure

pulmonary rehabilitation a programme of exercises and education aimed at reducing disability and handicap in chronic respiratory disease.

pulse oximetry a non-invasive method of assessing the amount of haemoglobin that is saturated with oxygen (*oxygen saturation*)

quality of life see *health status*

respiratory drive the stimulus to breathe. The main respiratory centre is in the medulla of the brain

respiratory failure failure to maintain oxygenation. It is usually taken to mean failure to maintain oxygenation above 8kPa

respiratory muscle training breathing exercises aimed at improving respiratory muscle strength and endurance. Its effectiveness in COPD is debatable

restrictive lung disease a disease that causes reduction in lung volumes (FVC and FEV_1) without reduction in flow rates through the airways (FEV_1/FVC ratio normal or high)

sarcoid an inflammatory disease of unknown cause affecting many parts of the body. Chronic sarcoidosis affecting the lungs causes diffuse fibrosis, reduction of lung volumes and, sometimes, airflow obstruction with air-trapping

shuttle walking test a method of assessing walking distance. The patient performs a paced walk between two points 10 metres apart (a shuttle) at an incrementally increasing pace, dictated by 'beeps' on a tape recording, until they are unable to maintain the pace

'silent area' a term used to describe the generation of airways 2–5mm in diameter. Considerable damage can occur in this area without causing symptoms

simple bronchitis chronic mucus production that is not associated with airflow obstruction

small airways disease pathological changes affecting airways 2–5mm in diameter, including occlusion of the airway with mucus, goblet cell hyperplasia, inflammatory changes in the airway wall, fibrosis and smooth muscle hypertrophy

smoking 'pack-years' a method of quantifying cigarette exposure:

$$\frac{\text{Number smoked per day}}{20} \times \text{Number of years smoked}$$

steroids see *corticosteroids*

theophyllines methylxanthine bronchodilator drug with a modest bronchodilator effect in COPD

total lung capacity (TLC) the volume of air in the lungs after maximum inhalation. It comprises the vital capacity and the residual volume

ultrasonic nebulisers nebulisers in which the aerosol is generated by agitating the nebuliser solution with ultrasonic vibrations produced by a piezo crystal

ventilation/perfusion mismatch a situation in which areas of the lung have a blood supply and no air and vice versa. It results in inefficient gas exchange

Venturi mask an oxygen mask that supplies a fixed percentage of oxygen

volume/time trace a graph produced by a spirometer whereby volume is plotted on the vertical axis and time on the horizontal axis

Useful addresses

Association of Respiratory Technology and Physiology
ARTP Administration
Suite 4 Sovereign House
Gate Lane
Boldmere
Birmingham B73 5TT
Tel/Fax: 0845 226 3062
Website: artp.org.uk
Runs training courses on respiratory function testing and assesses/certifies competence in the technique of spirometry

Breathe Easy Club
British Lung Foundation
73–75 Goswell Road
London EC1V 7ER
Tel: 020 7688 5555
Fax: 020 7688 5556
Website: www.lunguk.org
Self-help groups for social contact, support and encouragement

British Lung Foundation
73–75 Goswell Road
London EC1V 7ER
Tel: 020 7688 5555
Fax: 020 7688 5556
Website:
www.britishlungfoundation.com
Association of professionals who fund medical research and provide support and information to people with lung disease. Offers leaflets about suitable gentle exercises and breathing control

British Thoracic Society
17 Doughty Street
London WC1N 2PL
Tel: 020 7831 8778
Fax: 020 7831 8766
Website:
www.brit-thoracic.org.uk
Official body of medical practitioners, nurses, scientists and any professional with an interest in respiratory disease, promoting the interests of patients with lung diseases. For a copy of Spirometry in Practice see the website: www.brit-thoracic.org.uk/pdf/COPDSpirometryInPractice.pdf *or e-mail copd imc-group.co.uk or fax to 01252 845700*

Chest, Heart and Stroke Association (Northern Ireland)
21 Dublin Road
Belfast BT2 7HB
Tel: 028 90 320184
Fax: 028 90 333487
Website: www.nichsa.com
For information and advice

Chest, Heart and Stroke (Scotland)
65 North Castle Street
Edinburgh EH2 3LT
Tel: 0131 225 6963
Fax: 0131 220 6313
Website: www.chss.org.uk
For information and advice

Education for Health
The Athenaeum
10 Church Street
Warwick CV34 4AB
Tel: 01926 493313
Fax: 01926 493224
Website:
www.educationforhealth.org.uk
Courses on respiratory care for all health professionals.
Publications: Simply COPD, Simply Stop Smoking *and others*

Health Development Agency
Holborn Gate
330 High Holborn
London WC1V 7BA
Tel: 020 7430 0850
Fax: 020 7061 3390
Helpline: 0870 121 4194
Website: www.hda-online.org.uk
Formerly the Health Education Authority; it now deals only with research. Publications on health matters can be ordered via the Helpline

Quit (Smoking Quitlines)
England: 0800 00 22 00
Northern Ireland: 028 90 663 281
Scotland: 0800 84 84 84

Wales: 0800 169 0169 (national number)
Website: www.quit.org.uk
For help with trying to stop smoking

PCRS-UK
The Primary Care Respiratory Society
Smithy House
Waterbeck
Lockerbie DG11 3EY
Website: www.pcrs-uk.org

Royal College of Physicians of Edinburgh
9 Queen Street
Edinburgh EH2 1JQ
Tel: 0131 225 7324
Fax: 0131 220 3939
Website: www.rcpe.ac.uk/
Independent professional organisation promoting the highest standards in internal medicine

Addresses for breathlessness questionnaires

Chronic Respiratory Disease Index Questionnaire
Peggy Austin and Dr Holger Schünemann
Room 2C12
McMaster University Health Sciences Centre
Hamilton
Ontario L8N 3Z5
CANADA
Email: austinp mcmaster.ca
or schuneh mcmaster.ca

**St George's Respiratory
Questionnaire**
Professor Paul Jones
Division of Physiological
Medicine
St George's Hospital Medical
School
Cranmer Terrace
London SW17 0RE
Email: sadie sghms.ac.uk

**Breathing Problems
Questionnaire**
Professor Michael Hyland
Department of Psychology
University of Plymouth
Plymouth
Devon PL4 8AA
Email: mhyland plymouth.ac.uk

Manufacturers

Allen & Hanburys Ltd
Stockley Park West
Uxbridge
Middlesex UB11 1BT
Tel: 0800 221 441
Fax: 020 8990 4328
Website: www.gsk.com

AstraZeneca UK Ltd
Horizon Place
600 Capability Green
Luton
Bedfordshire LU1 3LU
Tel: 0800 7830 033
Fax: 01582 838003
Website: astrazeneca.co.uk

Aventis Pharma Ltd
Aventis House
50 Kings Hill Avenue
Kings Hill
West Malling
Kent ME19 4AH
Tel: 01732 584000
Fax: 01732 584080
Website: www.aventis.com

Boehringer Ingelheim Ltd
Ellesfield Avenue
Southern Industrial Estate
Bracknell
Berkshire RG12 8YS
Tel: 01344 424600
Fax: 01344 741444
Website:
www.boehringer-ingelheim.com

**Clement Clarke International
Ltd**
Unit A
Cartel Business Estate
Edinburgh Way
Harlow
Essex CM20 2TT
Tel: 01279 414969
Fax: 01279 456304
Website: www.clement-clarke.
com

Ferraris Medical Ltd
4 Harforde Court
John Tate Road
Hertford SG13 7NW
Tel: 01992 526300
Fax: 01992 526320
Website:
www.ferrarismedical.com

GlaxoSmithKline
Stockley Park West
Uxbridge
Middlesex UB11 1BT
Tel: 0800 221 441
Fax: 020 8990 4328
Website: www.gsk.com

IVAX Pharmaceuticals
Albert Basin
Armada Way
Royal Docks
London E16 2QJ
Tel: 08705 020304
Fax: 08705 323334
Website: www.ivax.co.uk

Micro Medical
Quayside
Chatham Maritime
Chatham
Kent ME4 4QY
Tel: 01634 893500
Fax: 01634 893600
Website: www.micromedical.co.uk

Napp Pharmaceuticals
Cambridge Science Park
Milton Road
Cambridge CB4 0GW
Tel: 01223 424444
Fax: 01223 424441
Website: www.napp.co.uk

Respironics Inc.
Profile Respiratory Systems
Heath Place
Bognor Regis
West Sussex PO22 9SL
Tel: 01243 840888
Fax: 01243 846100
Website: www.profilehs.com

Ranbaxy UK Ltd
6th floor
CP House
97–107 Uxbridge Road
London W5 5TL
Tel: 020 8280 1600
Fax: 020 8280 1616
Website: www.ranbaxy.com

Vitalograph Ltd
Maids Moreton
Buckingham MK18 1SW
Tel: 01280 827110
Fax: 01280 823302
Website: www.vitalograph.co.uk
Website: www.goldcopd.com
Recommends effective COPD management and prevention strategies for use in all countries. Gives the names and contact details of various national and international members of the group

Index

PRIORITY ORDER FORM

Cut out or photocopy this form and send it (post free in the UK) to:
Class Publishing Tel: 01256 302 699
FREEPOST 16705 Fax: 01256 812 558
Macmillan Distribution
Basingstoke RG21 6ZZ
Please send me urgently *Post included*
(tick below) price per copy (UK only)

☐	**Chronic Obstructive Pulmonary Disease in Primary Care** (ISBN 978 185969 225 0)	£20.99
☐	**COPD: Answers at your fingertips** (ISBN 978 1 85959 045 4)	£20.99
☐	**Vital Asthma** (ISBN 978 1 85959 107 9)	£20.99
☐	**Vital COPD** (ISBN 978 1 85959 114 7)	£20.99
☐	**Vital Lung Function** (ISBN 978 1 85959 161 1	£20.99
☐	**Heart Health: Answers at your fingertips** (ISBN 978 1 85959 157 4)	£20.99

TOTAL _____

Easy ways to pay

Cheque: I enclose a cheque payable to Class Publishing for £ _____

Credit card: Please debit my Mastercard ☐   Visa ☐   Amex ☐

Number _____   Expiry date _____

Name _____

My address for delivery is _____

Town _____ County _____ Postcode _____

Telephone number (*in case of query*) _____

Credit card billing address if different from above _____

Town _____ County _____ Postcode _____